Neurotrauma

NEUROSURGERY BY EXAMPLE:

Key Cases and Fundamental Principles
Series edited by: Nathan R. Selden, MD, PhD, FACS, FAAP

Neurotrauma

Edited by
Christopher J. Madden
Jack Jallo

OXFORD
UNIVERSITY PRESS

OXFORD
UNIVERSITY PRESS

Oxford University Press is a department of the University of Oxford. It furthers
the University's objective of excellence in research, scholarship, and education
by publishing worldwide. Oxford is a registered trade mark of Oxford University
Press in the UK and certain other countries.

Published in the United States of America by Oxford University Press
198 Madison Avenue, New York, NY 10016, United States of America.

CIP data is on file at the Library of Congress
ISBN 978–0–19–093625–9

9 8 7 6 5 4 3 2 1

Printed by Marquis, Canada

Contents

Series Editor's Preface

Dear Reader,

I am delighted to introduce this volume of *Neurosurgery by Example: Key Cases and Fundamental Principles*. Neurosurgical training and practice are based on managing a wide range of complex clinical cases with expert knowledge, sound judgment, and skilled technical execution. Our goal in this series is to present exemplary cases in the manner they are actually encountered in the neurosurgical clinic, hospital emergency department, and operating room.

In this volume, Drs. Christopher Madden and Jack Jallo invited a broad range of expert contributors to share their extensive wisdom and experience in all major areas of trauma neurosurgery. Each chapter contains a classic presentation of an important clinical entity, guiding readers through the assessment and planning, decision making, medical and surgical interventions, after care, and complication management. "Pivot points" illuminate the changes required to manage patients in alternate or atypical situations.

Each chapter also presents lists of "pearls" for the accurate diagnosis, successful treatment, and effective complication management of each clinical problem. These three focus areas will be especially helpful to neurosurgeons preparing to sit for the American Board of Neurological Surgery oral examination, which bases scoring on these three topics.

Finally, each chapter contains focused reviews of medical evidence and expected outcomes, helpful for counseling patients and setting accurate expectations. Rather than exhaustive reference lists, chapter authors provide focused lists of high-priority further reading recommended to deepen understanding. An additional chapter details the landscape of recent advances in multimodality monitoring.

The resulting volume should provide you with a dynamic tour through the practice of trauma neurosurgery, guided by some of the leading experts in North America. Additional volumes cover each subspecialty area of neurosurgery, using the same case-based approach and board review features.

—Nathan R. Selden, MD, PhD
Campagna Professor and Chair
Department of Neurological Surgery
Oregon Health & Science University

Contributors

Bizhan Aarabi, MD, FRCSC
Department of Neurosurgery
University of Maryland School of
   Medicine
Baltimore, MD

Fadi Alsaiegh, MD
Resident Physician
Department of Neurosurgery
Thomas Jefferson University Hospital
Philadelphia, PA

Kathleen R. Bell, MD
Professor, Chair
Kimberly Clark Distinguished Chair in
   Mobility Research
Department of Physical Medicine and
   Rehabilitation
University of Texas Southwestern
   Medical Center
Dallas, TX

Mitchell Couldwell, BS
Department of Neurosurgery, Clinical
   Neurosciences Center
University of Utah
Salt Lake City, UT

Tarek Y. El Ahmadieh, MD
Neurosurgical Resident
University of Texas Southwestern
   Medical Center
Dallas, TX

Ilyas Eli, MD
Department of Neurosurgery, Clinical
   Neurosciences Center
University of Utah
Salt Lake City, UT

James J. Evans, MD
Professor of Neurological Surgery and
   Otolaryngology
Department of Neurological Surgery
Thomas Jefferson University
Philadelphia, Pennsylvania, USA

Christopher J. Farrell, MD
Assistant Professor
Department of Neurological Surgery
Thomas Jefferson University
Philadelphia, PA

Evan Fitchett, BS
Sidney Kimmel Medical College at
   Thomas Jefferson University
Philadelphia, PA

Hermes Garcia, MD
Department of Neurosurgeon
Orlando Health Neuroscience and
   Rehabilitation Institute Neurosurgery
   Group
Orlando, FL

Tomas Garzon-Muvdi, MD, MSc.
Assistant professor of Neurosurgery
Department of Neurosurgery
UT Southwestern Medical Center
Dallas, Tx, USA

Ramesh Grandhi, MD
Department of Neurosurgery
  University of Utah Health
Salt Lake City, UT

Erin Graves, MD, Lt USN
Resident, Department of Neurological
  Surgery
Temple University, Lewis Katz School of
  Medicine
Philadelphia, PA

Patrick Greaney, MD
Department of General Surgery, Division
  of Plastic and Reconstructive Surgery
Thomas Jefferson University Hospital
Philadelphia, PA

Gregory W. J. Hawryluk, MD, PhD
Departments of Neurosurgery and
  Neurology, University of Utah Health
Salt Lake City, UT

Sara Hefton, MD
Assistant Professor of Neurology and
  Neurosurgery
Thomas Jefferson University
Philadelphia, PA

**Adel Helmy, MB BChir, PhD,
  FRCS (SN)**
Division of Neurosurgery, Department of
  Clinical Neurosciences
Addenbrooke's Hospital
Cambridge, UK

Zachary L. Hickman, MD
Department of Neurosurgery, Icahn
  School of Medicine at Mount Sinai and
  NYC Health + Hospitals/Elmhurst
New York, NY

**Peter J. A. Hutchinson, MBBS, PhD,
  FRCS (SN), FmedSci**
Division of Neurosurgery, Department of
  Clinical Neurosciences
Addenbrooke's Hospital
Cambridge, UK

Brandon Isaacson, MD
University of Texas Southwestern
  Medical Center
Dallas, TX

Jack Jallo, MD, PhD
Professor of Neurological Surgery,
  Division Director of Neuro-Trauma
  and Critical Care
Department of Neurosurgery
Thomas Jefferson University Hospital
Philadelphia, PA

Hongzhao Ji, MD
University of Texas Southwestern
  Medical Center
Dallas, TX

Benjamin Kafka, MD
Resident, Department of Neurological
  Surgery
University of Texas Southwestern
  Medical Center
Dallas, TX

Lydia Kaoutzani, MD
Division of Neurosurgery, Beth Israel
  Deaconess Medical Center
Harvard Medical School
Boston, MA

Omaditya Khanna, MD
Resident Physician
Department of Neurological Surgery
Thomas Jefferson University Hospital
Philadelphia, PA. USA.

**Abdelhakim Khellaf, MDCM
  Candidate**
Division of Neurosurgery, Department of
  Clinical Neurosciences
Addenbrooke's Hospital
Cambridge, UK

Ryan S. Kitagawa, MD
Department of Neurosurgery
University of Texas Health
  Sciences Center
Houston, TX

Cole T. Lewis
Department of Neurosurgery
University of Texas Health
    Sciences Center
Houston, TX

Christopher J. Madden, MD
Professor, Department of Neurological
    Surgery
University of Texas Southwestern
    Medical Center
Dallas, TX

Konstantinos Margetis, MD, PhD
Department of Neurosurgery, Icahn
    School of Medicine at Mount Sinai and
    NYC Health + Hospitals/Elmhurst
New York, NY

Amy A. Mathews, MD
Assistant Professor, Department of
    Physical Medicine and Rehabilitation
University of Texas Southwestern
    Medical Center
Dallas, TX

Benjamin McGahan, MD
Department of Neurological Surgery
The Ohio State University Wexner
    Medical Center
Columbus, OH

John McGregor, MD
Department of Neurological Surgery
The Ohio State University Wexner
    Medical Center
Columbus, OH

Mark A. Miller, MD, DMD
Department of Oral and Maxillofacial
    Surgery
University of Texas Health San Antonio
San Antonio, TX

Geoffrey Peitz, MD
Department of Neurosurgery
University of Texas Health San Antonio
San Antonio, TX

Courtney Pendleton
Department of Neurosurgery
    Thomas Jefferson University Hospital
Philadelphia, PA

Aaron R. Plitt, MD
Resident, Department of Neurological
    Surgery
University of Texas Southwestern
    Medical Center
Dallas, TX

Craig H. Rabb, MD
Department of Neurosurgery, Clinical
    Neurosciences Center
University of Utah
Salt Lake City, UT

Kim Rickert, MD
Associate Professor of Surgery, Division
    of Neurosurgery
Geisinger Commonwealth School of
    Medicine
Sayre, PA

**Richard B. Rodgers, MD,
    FAANS, FACS**
Associate Professor of Clinical
    Neurosurgery
Indiana University School
    of Medicine
Goodman Campbell
    Brain and Spine
Indianapolis, IN

Richard F. Schmidt, MD
Resident
Department of Neurological
    Surgery
Thomas Jefferson University
Philadelphia, PA, USA

Varun Shah, BS
Department of Neurological
    Surgery
The Ohio State University Wexner
    Medical Center
Columbus, OH

Martina Stippler, MD, FAANS
Division of Neurosurgery, Beth Israel
  Deaconess Medical Center
Harvard Medical School
Boston, MA

Thana N. Theofanis, MD
Department of Neurological Surgery
Thomas Jefferson University Hospital
Philadelphia, PA

Shelly D. Timmons, MD, PhD
Professor of Neurological Surgery
Pennsylvania State University
State College, PA 16801,
United States

Nathaniel Toop, MD
Department of Neurological Surgery
The Ohio State University Wexner
  Medical Center
Columbus, OH

Philip A. Villanueva, MD
Director Neurotrauma and Neurosurgical
  Critical Care
Temple University/Lewis Katz School of
  Medicine
Philadelphia, PA

Mohamed A. Zaazoue, MD, MSc
Department of Neurological Surgery
Indiana University School of Medicine
Indianapolis, IN

Hussein A. Zeineddine
Department of Neurosurgery
University of Texas Health
  Sciences Center
Houston, TX

Neurotrauma

Medical Management of Elevated Intracranial Pressure

Courtney Pendleton and Jack Jallo

Case Presentation

A 24-year-old man fell approximately 30 feet while working as a roofer; he had a loss of consciousness following the impact but regained consciousness and was agitated and able to protect his airway during transport via EMS to a level one trauma center.

On arrival, his exam had deteriorated, and he arrived with a Glasgow Coma Scale (GCS) score of 6T. He was intubated on arrival in the emergency department trauma bay. His initial exam demonstrated multiple facial and scalp lacerations and abrasions, along with ecchymosis and edema surrounding the right orbit requiring lateral canthotomy. His pupils were 4 mm and sluggish bilaterally, he had cough and gag reflexes and a left corneal reflex; he withdrew all extremities to pain.

Questions

1. What is the most likely diagnosis?
2. What imaging should be obtained emergently?
3. What imaging should be obtained in a nonurgent fashion?

Assessment and Planning

Given the nature of his injury, the presence of multiple lacerations and ecchymoses, and the poor neurological exam, a significant intracranial hemorrhage was suspected. The patient was taken for an emergent noncontrast CT of the head and cervical spine. Additional trauma scans of the chest, abdomen, and pelvis with reconstructions of the thoracolumbar spine were also obtained as part of the trauma protocol.

The head CT demonstrated multiple facial fractures, a nondisplaced linear skull fracture, frontal sinus fracture, left side subdural hemorrhage, bilateral frontal intraparenchymal contusions, and subarachnoid hemorrhage (Figure 1.1).

A CT angiogram (CTA) of the head and neck was obtained during the same scanning period because the patient remained hemodynamically stable. The scan showed no evidence of aneurysm, dissection, or vascular malformation.

In cases where the patient's exam is out of proportion to the extent of intracranial injury seen on head CT, a noncontrast MRI brain may provide additional information, particularly regarding diffuse axonal injury (DAI), that clarifies prognosis and may

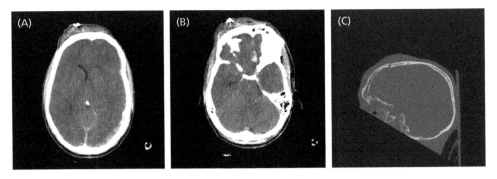

Figure 1.1 (A) Anteroposterior plain skull film, and (B&C) Axial CT brain showing left occipital skull fracture extending down to suboccipital bone.

inform family discussions and treatment planning. However, MRI is not recommended as an emergent imaging modality.

Questions

1. How do these radiographic findings influence the treatment plan?
2. What interventions should be performed immediately for this patient?
3. What additional interventions may be considered prior to surgical intervention?

Oral Boards Review: Diagnostic Pearls

- On plain head CT, thoroughly assess bone, parenchyma, and ventricles for pathology.
  - Mass lesions, midline shift, displaced or comminuted skull fractures are reason to consider immediate operative management.
- All suspicious lesions, particularly in young patients, should have additional vascular imaging obtained.
  - CTA head and neck can assess for arteriovenous malformation (AVM), aneurysm, and dissections.
  - MR angiogram is not useful as an emergent study in an unstable patient.
- In patients with an exam out of proportion to injury on head CT:
  - Consider an MRI when able to assess for DAI.
  - Imaging of the craniocervical junction, cervical spine, and thoracolumbar spine may uncover other causes for a poor exam.

Decision Making

Although his imaging demonstrated multicompartment hemorrhages, there was no significant midline shift or evidence of mass effect. Therefore plans were made for medical management of his injuries. The patient was admitted to the neurosurgical intensive care unit (NICU). The Brain Trauma Foundation (BTF) guidelines previously recommended intracranial pressure (ICP) monitoring in patients with GCS of less than 8 and an abnormal head CT, or patients with a normal head CT if they had two or more of the inclusion criteria: age older than 40, motor posturing, SBP less than 90 mm Hg. While these characteristics frequently describe the majority of patients who receive ICP monitoring at our institution, the most recent BTF guidelines removed these criteria as the relevant studies did not meet evidence standards. The only recommendation for monitoring is currently that ICP monitoring may reduce in-hospital and 2-week mortality.

The gold standard ICP monitor is an external ventriculostomy (EVD), and the BTF guidelines emphasize that these are favored because they allow for monitoring and treatment of ICP via CSF drainage, and they can be recalibrated, unlike other available monitors. The recommendation is to treat ICP of more than 22 mm Hg because ICP above this threshold is associated with increased mortality.

Prior to any procedures, it is imperative that a full set of labs be checked to ensure platelets and coagulation markers are within normal limits. If possible, a medication history should be obtained specifically asking about antiplatelet and anticoagulation agents. Appropriate reversal agents should be administered as needed. In addition, any patient with concern for elevated ICP should have a chem 7, full electrolyte panel, and serum osmolality drawn on admission to aid treatment planning.

The location of EVD placement requires additional consideration in patients with traumatic injuries or fractures. In general, we prefer right-sided ventriculostomies to minimize disruption of eloquent cortex. In cases with significant left-side hemorrhage or injury, we consider an ipsilateral EVD to avoid further injury should a peri-catheter hemorrhage arise.

Patients undergoing medical management of elevated ICPs should have central venous access and arterial lines placed to allow administration of medication and maintenance of blood pressure goals in accordance with BTF guidelines (SBP >100 patients 50–69, >110 for patients 15–49 and >70). Consideration may be given to placement of a Swan-Ganz catheter in patients who require barbiturate coma for ICP management.

Following placement of the EVD, the patient's ICPs were noted to be 25–30 despite drainage of CSF. Additional medical interventions were begun. Short-term temporizing approaches include hyperventilation to decrease P_{CO_2} and sitting the patient upright. These interventions should be instituted while additional medications are being obtained and should not be used as the sole means of addressing persistently elevated ICP. The only recommendation in the 4th edition BTF guidelines regarding hyperventilation is Level IIb, that prolonged prophylactic hyperventilation is not recommended. Previous editions specifically recommended hyperventilation as a temporizing measure. While this recommendation was removed because it was based on literature that did not meet inclusion criteria for the 4th edition (case series only), it may still be a useful temporizing measure while medications are being obtained or operative intervention is being arranged.

The benefit of ICP monitoring via an EVD includes the ability to drain CSF for management of elevated ICP: the available guidelines are Level III recommendations that continuous drainage via an EVD zeroed at the midbrain may be more effective than intermittent drainage and that CSF drainage may be considered in patients with GCS of less than 6 in the first 24 h. This is a new topic in the 4th edition of the guidelines, and additional high-quality studies are needed to enable more thorough recommendations in future editions.

The most recent BTF guidelines state that while hyperosmolar therapy may decrease ICP, there is insufficient evidence to recommend a specific agent (i.e., mannitol, hypertonic saline) for this therapy. Earlier editions of the guidelines stated that mannitol in doses of 0.25–1 g/kg was effective in reducing ICP and recommended using mannitol either in patients with evidence of elevated ICP on intracranial monitor or in patients with clinical evidence of herniation syndromes or progressive neurological deficit.

Pharmaceutical methods of treating elevated ICP include intermittent boluses of narcotics (our institution frequently uses fentanyl), continuous drip of these medications, continuous drip of sedating agents (i.e., Precedex, propofol), or the use of barbiturates to induce burst suppression on EEG for intractable ICPs. Level IIb recommendations suggest barbiturate-induced burst suppression should not be used prophylactically but may be used for refractory ICP provided hemodynamic stability is maintained. Propofol is recommended for control of ICP, with the caveat that it does not improve mortality or 6-month outcomes. In patients being treated with high-dose propofol for ICP management, it is important to monitor creatinine, creatinine kinase, and clinical signs of renal function to ensure that propofol infusion syndrome (PRIS), which carries a high mortality rate in itself, does not occur.

The BTF guidelines do not recommend prophylactic hypothermia; however, hypothermia remains an option in the ICP management pathway for patients with refractory elevated ICP. Hypothermia may be achieved with cutaneous cooling pads or via a central venous catheter system. Central access may minimize shivering but does not obviate it. Our protocol is to begin by cooling patients to 35°C, using BuSpar and magnesium continuous infusions as prophylaxis against shivering. In patients who develop significant shivering, we attempt counter-warming with heated air blankets (i.e., Bair Hugger). If this fails, and if shivering affects ICP management, a paralytic infusion such as rocuronium is strongly considered. Of note, patients with severe shivering at 35°C may be cooled to 33°C, which minimizes the physiologic shivering response. Patients who are undergoing therapeutic hypothermia treatment, who do not have clinical shivering, but continue to have elevated ICPs, may be having micro-shivering and may also benefit from a paralytic. During hypothermia, the physiologic response is to force potassium intracellularly, leading to hypokalemia on daily lab checks. However, as rewarming will reverse this process, we recommend judicious repletion of potassium in these patients, with a goal around 2.5–3.0 provided there are no EKG changes, to avoid severe hyperkalemia upon rewarming.

Surgical Procedure

The details of operative intervention for intractable increased ICP are described in a separate chapter.

Operative intervention should be considered in patients where medical treatment options for elevated ICP (as detailed in the prior section) have been exhausted and in patients where imaging demonstrates clear mass effect/midline shift. It is imperative that the treating neurosurgeon and critical care teams be familiar with all medical treatment options and that consideration is given to how far along the pathway (hypothermia, barbiturate coma, etc.) they want to proceed before operative intervention is offered.

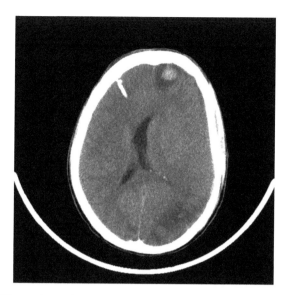

Figure 1.2 (A&B) Axial CT brain showing large left occipital/suboccipital epidural hematoma with mass effect.

It is likewise paramount that frank conversations are had with the patient's family and decision makers. The patient's age, general medical condition, extent of intracranial injury, and presence of other injuries are all important factors to consider when discussing prognosis, goals of care, and surgical intervention.

In our patient, we discussed at length with his family that despite aggressive medical management, his ICP remained high, and, given the evolution of his intracranial injury on repeat head CT (Figure 1.2), we recommended a decompressive hemicraniectomy as our next treatment option. In our conversations with any patient's family, we stress that operative intervention is designed to reduce the risk of mortality but may not effect overall functional prognosis or neurological recovery. The BTF guidelines specify that bifrontal craniectomies do not improve outcomes but successfully reduce ICP and lead to decreased ICU stay; frontotemporoparietal craniectomies deompressive hemicraniectomy (DHC) more than 15 cm diameter reduce mortality and may improve neurological outcomes.

Oral Boards Review: Management Pearls

- Traumatic injury causing clear mass effect, midline shift, or depressed skull fracture requiring repair should be managed with initial surgical intervention. Intraoperative placement of an ICP monitor should be considered.
- Escalating medical management using CSF drainage, temporizing measures, hyperosmolar therapy, sedation, and barbiturate coma should be considered.
- PRIS is a potentially fatal complication. Long-term high-dose propofol should be avoided; renal function should be monitored during treatment course.
- Early and frequent family discussions should occur. The mortality rate and neurological prognosis should be frankly described. Patient condition, age, and other injuries should be considered.

> • Surgical intervention requires clear communication between the surgeon, operating room team, and anesthesia team. Adequate equipment and supplies should be confirmed; complications or intraoperative emergencies should be anticipated and clearly communicated to entire team along with a contingency plan.

Aftercare

Immediately postoperatively, patients require close monitoring of ICP to ensure it does not remain elevated. We consider weaning hyperosmolar therapy in this period provided there are no ongoing issues with ICP.

Nursing staff, critical care team, and house staff should be educated regarding the status of the hemicraniectomy flap at the conclusion of the case, to have a baseline for future evaluations. We recommend having all team members assess the patient after return from the operating room.

Slow reversal of sedating agents should be planned, with close monitoring of hemodynamic status, cEEG, and ICP. There should be contingency plans for re-escalating medical management if elevated ICPs recur. It is imperative these plans be consistently communicated between the surgeon, critical care team, house staff, and any night-float/weekend coverage/on-call teams.

> **Pivot Points**
>
> • The initial head CT should be assessed for surgical lesion. If this is present, initial management should be operative. If not, consider ICP monitor, and medical management for ICP of more than 22 mm Hg.
> • Early family discussions should focus on course of care and interest in operative management. If family does not want to pursue surgery, exhaustive medical therapy, included barbiturate coma and hypothermia, should be considered. If family wants surgery, consider a contingency plan for what point in escalating medical management will prompt a trip to the operating room.
> • Although the BTF guidelines have changed, the 3rd edition criteria for ICP monitoring may be considered in determining which patients require ICP monitoring and which may be observed via clinical exam. If the patient has GCS of less than 8 and an abnormal head CT, or a normal head CT but meets two or more of the criteria (age older than 40, motor posturing, SBP less than 90 mm Hg), it is reasonable to consider a monitor. If the patient has GCS of greater than 8, monitoring exam with minimal sedation remains an option.

Complications and Management

Medical management options are not without complications. Hyperosmolar therapy with mannitol can lead to hypotension, while hypertonic saline may lead to cardiac arrhythmias and renal dysfunction. Vasopressors required to maintain goal SBP or mean arterial pressure (MAP) while patients are receiving hyperosmolar therapy, sedation, or barbiturate-induced burst suppression may cause peripheral vascular constriction with injury to extremities; if peripheral IVs are used, infiltration can cause compartment syndrome, tissue necrosis, and limb loss.

Patients with high-dose sedation needs may demonstrate hypotension and bradycardia (particularly with Precedex). High-dose propofol may lead to PRIS with potentially fatal results. Avoiding doses of more than 4 mg/kg/h for more than 24 h is recommended. Daily checks of triglycerides, creatinine/BUN, and creatinine kinase may catch PRIS early.

In patients requiring barbiturate-induced burst suppression, complications may arise when discussing end-of-life care, particularly in patients in whom progression to brain death is suspected or whose families wish to pursue organ donation options. The half-life of phenobarbital or pentobarbital, the most commonly used long-acting barbiturates in our institution, is 50–120 h. Drug level testing is available but is often sent to outside facilities, and it may take days to obtain a result. While barbiturates may be necessary for managing intractable ICPs, in families who are considering organ donation, a discussion about the challenges of these medications in assessing brain death may be beneficial.

Central venous access is recommended for patients requiring medical management of elevated ICPs, but these lines may lead to infection, fistula formation, accidental cannulization of an artery, hemo/pneumothorax, nerve injuries, or air emboli during line removal.

Hypothermic therapy may be achieved through central cooling catheters or cutaneous cooling pads. Central catheters carry the risks of line placement. Cutaneous cooling pads may limit the patient's ability to undergo scans (i.e., MRIs, lower extremity ultrasound for deep venous thrombosis screening), and can cause skin breakdown and frostbite. In extreme cases tissue damage requires management with hyperbaric oxygen and management in specialized burn centers. Frequent skin checks, particularly in patients with consistently low water-bath temperatures, are necessary to avoid serious injury.

The placement of an ICP monitor or EVD may lead to superficial skin infection, meningitis, or ventriculitis; despite best efforts, already injured brain is friable, and there is a risk of worsening, possibly life-ending intracranial or intraventricular hemorrhage following the procedure.

Infections in general are best managed through avoidance: proper sterile technique, limiting staff in the room, hair clipping when applicable, and clean dressings. There remains controversy surrounding the benefit of administering prophylactic antibiotics during bedside ventriculostomy procedures. While continued antibiotic coverage is not recommended, a single peri-procedure dose of antibiotics to cover skin flora may reduce the rate of ventriculostomy-associated infections.

Postoperatively, wound dehiscence is a potential complication, often exacerbated by patients who have limited ability to change position, where the hemicraniectomy site (other than bifrontal) may remain dependent, particularly the posterior-inferior aspect. Frequent repositioning, including using blankets or foam pillows to off-load the posterior scalp and maintain head rotation in alternating directions may help alleviate the problem. Daily wound checks are essential, and good communication with family members and potential rehabilitation or skill nursing facility staff regarding positioning needs and wound care may help catch any breakdown early.

> ### Oral Boards Review: Complication Pearls
>
> - Infections are serious complications of central lines, EVDs, and surgery. Avoidance is the best management. Sterile technique, limiting room traffic, and peri-procedure antibiotics help mitigate the risk.
> - Frequent skin checks for patients with cutaneous cooling pads for hypothermia may help avoid serious skin breakdown and tissue damage.
> - Postoperatively, close attention to off-loading pressure on the incision, frequent repositioning, and daily wound checks minimize the risk of dehiscence and infection.

Evidence and Outcomes

The BTF offer mostly Level II and III recommendations for medical and surgical management of ICP. The only Level I recommendation is the avoidance of steroids.

While hyperosmolar therapy is widely used for ICP management, there remains no clear evidence what agent is most effective at addressing ICP or at reducing mortality.

Severe traumatic brain injury (TBI) with elevated ICP remains a significant issue for neurosurgeons and critical care physicians. While there are many case series and retrospective studies regarding management, there are few high-quality prospective studies assessing the ability of medical and operative interventions to reduce mortality, reduce ICU and overall hospital stay, or improve functional outcomes.

Further Reading

Carney N, Totten AM, O'Reilly C. Guidelines for the management of severe traumatic brain injury. *Neurosurgery*. 2017 Jan 1;80(1):6–15.

Chesnut RM, Temkin N, Carney N, et al. Global Neurotrauma Research Group. A trial of intracranial-pressure monitoring in traumatic brain injury. *NEJM*. 2012 Dec 27;367(26):2471–2481.

Hutchinson PJ, Kolias AG, Timofeev IS, et al. RESCUEicp Trial Collaborators. Trial of decompressive craniectomy for traumatic intracranial hypertension. *NEJM*. 2016 Sept 22;375(12):1119–1130.

Surgical Treatment of Raised Intracranial Pressure

Mohamed A. Zaazoue and Richard B. Rodgers

2

Case Presentation

A 32-year-old previously healthy male patient presented to our emergency department (ED) after being struck by a car while trying to get into his own vehicle. Per bystanders, the patient was thrown several feet away. He was combative at the scene, with altered mental status, and therefore was intubated for airway protection by EMS responders. EMS staff reported decorticate posturing en route to the ED. On examination by the neurosurgeon in the ED, patient had a Glasgow Coma Scale (GCS) score of 7T, localizing with both upper extremities in response to pain and withdrawing to pain in both lower extremities. His right pupil was 4 mm and left pupil was 2 mm, both sluggishly reactive to light. He had a large stellate laceration with contamination over the right temporoparietal region of the scalp.

As a part of the trauma surgery team's evaluation, the patient underwent CT imaging of the head. This head CT (Figure 2.1A,B) revealed a right middle fossa epidural hematoma with associated skull fracture, contrecoup left cortical contusions, and mild effacement of the basal cisterns.

Questions

1. What are the first-line management steps for an unresponsive patient presenting to the ED?
2. What are the components of the GCS?
3. In an unresponsive patient, what is the most appropriate diagnostic modality to assess: (a) traumatic brain injury, (b) cervical spine injury?

Assessment and Planning

The patient suffered a significant head trauma with severe traumatic brain injury (TBI). Clinical signs of raised intracranial pressure (ICP) included diminished level of consciousness, a period of decorticate posturing, and unequal pupils. His head CT suggested elevated ICP as well, with a mass lesion (epidural hematoma), contrecoup contusions, and effacement of cisterns. Patient's head was kept elevated in bed and he was given a bolus dose of hypertonic saline for presumed elevated ICP. He was taken emergently to the operating room for evacuation of the epidural hematoma. Due to the complex

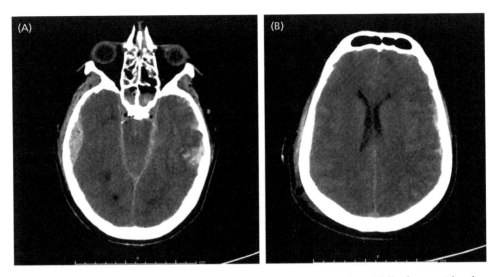

Figure 2.1 Non-contrast, axial CT of the head showing a right middle fossa epidural hematoma with associated skull fracture (A), contrecoup left cortical contusions (A), and mild effacement of the basal cisterns (B).

laceration and contamination of fractures, bone was not replaced. A right-sided external ventricular drain (EVD) was also placed through a separate incision and was kept open at 10 mm Hg above the level of the external auditory meatus. Postoperatively, patient was taken to the ICU, where he was kept on continuous IV sedation using propofol and fentanyl.

Over the ensuing days, the patient's neurological examination gradually declined, and his ICP trended upward. Nonsurgical measures to control ICP, including head elevation, sedation, osmotic therapy, and CSF drainage failed. Neurotelemetry was performed to rule out evidence of seizures.

Oral Boards Review: Diagnostic Pearls

- Physical examination, including the GCS, is crucial to assess TBI patients and determine their management plan.
  - Unresponsive patients are initially managed using the standard approach of priorities: Airway, Breathing, and Circulation. For patients with GCS of 8 or less, endotracheal intubation for airway protection is required.
  - Patients with GCS of 8 or less and CT revealing structural brain injury should undergo ICP monitoring.
  - Focal neurological deficits such as unequal pupils or hemiparesis may be caused by a unilateral mass effect and impending brain herniation.
- Head CT is the first-line diagnostic imaging to exclude intracranial abnormalities.
- To exclude cervical spine injuries, clinical examination and x-ray are usually sufficient for responsive patients. For symptomatic or unresponsive patients, a CT cervical spine is needed to exclude injury.

Decision Making

Follow-up imaging revealed worsening left-to-right midline shift and compressed cisterns (Figure 2.2A,B). Decision was made to take the patient back to the operating room, this time for a left-sided craniectomy to better control the raised ICP. Postoperatively, the ICP was controlled at less than 20 mm Hg, and, over the next few days, the patient began to show neurological improvement. Trials to wean the EVD failed, so the patient was taken to the operating room for ventriculoperitoneal shunt (VPS) placement.

Five weeks post-injury, patient was discharged to a rehabilitation facility. On neurological examination, he was opening his eyes to verbal stimulation, producing sounds (tracheostomized), and was following commands with all extremities. Three and a half months post-injury, patient underwent a left cranioplasty procedure, done using his bone flap that was removed during the second craniectomy surgery. He is now back home with his family. His only deficit is mild word-finding difficulty.

ICP Monitoring

Neurosurgeons are typically involved early in the management of TBI patients, usually starting during the ED stay. Patients with altered mental status are commonly intubated on scene or shortly after arriving in the ED for airway protection and/or ventilation. Sedatives and paralytics used during airway intubation interfere with the neurological

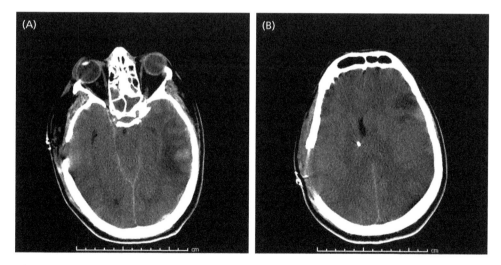

Figure 2.2 Non-contrast, axial CT of the head showing post-operative changes after a right temporoparietal craniectomy for evacuation of epidural hematoma (A and B) and placement of a right-sided external ventricular drain (B).

examination, so ideally this exam takes place prior to administration of these medications. However, definitive airway protection should not be delayed in the unstable patient.

Indications: There is no Level I or IIa evidence to support ICP monitoring. Level IIb evidence shows that ICP monitoring can help reduce in-hospital and 2-week post-injury mortality. Nevertheless, the Brain Trauma Foundation still supports the following indications for ICP monitor placement:

- GCS of 8 or less and an abnormal CT scan (including hematomas, contusions, swelling, herniation, or compressed basal cisterns)
- TBI patients with a normal CT scan if two or more of the following features are present: age older than 40 years, systolic blood pressure of less than 90 mm Hg, or motor posturing

Surgical procedure: Whenever decision is made that a TBI patient requires ICP monitoring, the surgical procedure should be done without delay. The only exception is in patients with severe bleeding tendencies or coagulopathies. If informed consent can't be obtained from a family member, an emergent consent is usually signed in the ED by two physicians. At our institution, parenchymal ICP monitors are placed at bedside. Generally, right frontal ICP monitor placement is preferred, but this can be individualized based on the patient's particular injury and potential need for further surgical interventions. A twist drill is used to create a hole at Kocher's point (10–11 cm from the nasion and 2–3 cm from the midline). Opening ICP should be noted to help guide further management. Treatment should be initiated for ICP of greater than 22 mm Hg. ICP monitoring can be discontinued if the pressures are normal for 24–48 h.

Questions

1. What is the upper limit of normal range of ICP in a supine, healthy adult?
2. What are the anatomic landmarks of Kocher's point?

Surgical Management

For patients with uncontrolled elevation of ICP, there are three surgical interventions that neurosurgeons can offer:

1. EVD placement
2. Evacuation of mass lesion
3. Decompressive craniectomy (unilateral or bifrontal)

External Ventricular Drain Placement

EVD can be used for simultaneous ICP monitoring and CSF drainage. CSF drainage, especially in patients with hydrocephalus, can help lower elevated ICP by decreasing the volume occupied by CSF within the closed cranial compartment. Current evidence in the literature supports continuous drainage over intermittent drainage for ICP control. The rate and extent of drainage should be guided by the ICP value. Changing the height of the EVD in relation to the external auditory meatus (EAM) can alter the rate of drainage. At the EAM, which is approximately the same level as the foramen of Monroe, the EVD is considered to be set at 0. Antimicrobial-impregnated catheters help reduce catheter-related infections.

Indications: For patients with hydrocephalus, it is preferred to place an EVD initially and use it for both monitoring and treating ICP. In a tiered management protocol, EVD placement can be an early surgical intervention used to control persistently elevated ICP as measured by a parenchymal probe.

Surgical procedure: Similar to ICP monitor placement, an EVD can be placed through the Kocher's point, and the catheter is tunneled to exit away from the entry point. A larger twist drill bit, or even a burr hole drill, is used to create a wider hole in the skull than the one typically used for ICP monitors because of the larger diameter of the catheter compared to that of the cranial access bolt and intraparenchymal ICP monitor.

Evacuation of Mass Lesion

There are different mass lesions that can develop as sequelae of TBI. The most efficient initial diagnostic tool to detect such lesions is a CT scan of the head without contrast. These lesions can cause direct compression on vital neurological centers in the brain leading to neurological deficits or deteriorating neurological examination.

Indications for prompt evacuation of mass lesions:

- Extradural hematoma (EDH): Hematomas greater than 30 cm³ should be surgically evacuated regardless of the patient's GCS score. Patients with EDH of less than 30 cm³ who are comatose (GCS ≤8) and/or with unequal pupils should also undergo prompt surgical evacuation of hematoma. Conservative management with serial CT scanning and close neurological observation can be done if all the following criteria are met: EDH less than 30 cm³, thickness of less than 15 mm, midline shift of less than 5 mm, GCS of greater than 8 and no focal neurological deficit.

- Acute subdural hematoma (SDH): Hematomas with greater than 10 mm thickness or midline shift greater than 5 mm require surgical evacuation. For patients with smaller SDH who are either comatose (GCS ≤8), or with unequal pupils, or who have an ICP of greater than 20 mm Hg, surgery should also be considered.

- Intraparenchymal hematomas: Surgery to evacuate intraparenchymal hematoma should be considered if there is CT evidence of perilesional mass effect, focal neurological deficit, or ICP elevation refractory to nonsurgical management.

- Frontal and temporal lobe contusions: Patients with contusions of greater than 50 cm³ in volume, or patients with GCS of 8 or less, with a midline shift of greater than 5 mm and a contusion of greater than 20 cm³ might benefit from surgery.

- Posterior fossa lesions: The threshold to evacuate posterior fossa mass lesions should be lower due to the possibility of direct compression of the brainstem or the fourth ventricle, which may lead to hydrocephalus. Patients with poor GCS score or neurological deficit referable to the lesion should be considered for surgical evacuation.

Surgical procedure: Surgical evacuation of mass lesions is typically performed using a craniotomy appropriate for lesion location, with replacement of the bone flap at the end of the procedure.

Decompressive Craniectomy

The skull is a closed compartment that is occupied by brain, blood, and CSF. When ICP elevations in the closed compartment are refractory to medical treatment and CSF diversion, an option in management is to perform a decompressive craniectomy (i.e., open the compartment) to create more room in the cranial cavity by removing a large portion of the skull. Decompressive craniectomy can be primary, when the bone flap is not replaced at the time of surgery for evacuation of an intracranial hematoma. Secondary craniectomy occurs when the procedure is performed as part of a tiered management protocol for ICP control in TBI patients in order to ensure adequate cerebral perfusion pressure. Literature shows that decompressive craniectomy can lower the mortality rates of TBI patients. However, it is important to note that this improvement in survival may come at the expense of a higher rate of patients with vegetative states or significant disabilities or dependence compared to patients who did not undergo decompressive craniectomy. Such patients would have otherwise not survived their significant TBI had they not received this procedure. Therefore, it is necessary to properly counsel patients' families about the possible outcomes and expectations of decompressive craniectomy in order to allow them reach an informed decision regarding the treatment of the TBI patient.

Indications: Assuming any mass lesion has been addressed, first-tier management includes head of bed elevation, sedation/analgesia, and intermittent ventricular drainage (if EVD placed initially). Second-tier management includes continuous ventricular drainage, hyperosmolar therapy (hypertonic saline or mannitol), and mild hyperventilation (pco_2 30–35 mm Hg). Third-tier therapies include decompressive craniectomy, continuous paralytic administration, and barbiturate coma. It should be noted that despite their common use in neurosurgical practice, there is a scarcity of Level I evidence supporting recommendations for these measures regarding ICP control. In some institutions, decompressive craniectomy is considered when ICP levels are greater than 25 mm Hg for more than 1–12 h.

Surgical technique: Decompressive craniectomy can be unilateral frontotemporoparietal (also known as hemicraniectomy) or bifrontal. Hemicraniectomy is indicated when local mass effect (e.g., from an acute subdural hematoma) and/or midline shift is noted. In this case, the hemicraniectomy is performed on the side of the mass effect (i.e., opposite to the direction of the midline shift). The hemicraniectomy should be wide enough (not less than 12 × 15 cm or ≥15 cm in diameter), extending basally into the temporal skull base to adequately lower the elevated ICP and decompress the cerebral hemisphere, including the temporal lobe, thus decreasing the risk of herniation. Bifrontal craniectomy is typically performed in patients with bifrontal contusions with swelling and can also be utilized in patients with diffuse, nonfocal brain swelling. The dura is incised to further provide room for the swollen brain. Duraplasty is then performed using either autologous graft (pericranium or fascia lata) or synthetic dura substitutes. Regardless of the material used for dural repair, it is not always necessary to suture the dura in a watertight fashion, especially if the brain is actively swelling, thus necessitating prompt closure to avoid herniation and compression across the sharp bony edges of the craniectomy. The bone flap can be stored in a freezer according to hospital-specific protocols or placed in the abdominal subcutaneous tissue if such storage resources are not available or there is a fear patient will be lost to follow-up.

Complications: Common complications include posttraumatic hydrocephalus and subdural hygroma, with or without hemorrhagic transformation. Contralateral subdural or epidural hematoma may occur. *Syndrome of the trephined* has been reported in patients who underwent craniectomy. It is characterized by headaches, confusion, memory loss, mood disturbances, and even motor deficits in the form of contralateral upper limb weakness not previously caused by the TBI. This syndrome can usually be reversed by cranioplasty.

Cranioplasty

Following recovery from elevated ICP, cranioplasty should be performed for cosmetic purposes, as well as for potential neurological benefit. The procedure is usually performed weeks to months after the original trauma to allow time for wound healing and TBI recovery. It can be done using the patient's autologous bone flap or prosthetic material made of titanium or plastic polymers.

Oral Boards Review: Management Pearls

- If a TBI patient needs ICP monitoring, it should be placed without delay. The procedure can be done at bedside in the ED or the ICU. Right frontal location is generally preferred.
- Treatment is needed if ICP is greater than 22 mm Hg. ICP management is a tiered approach, with early tiers including head of bed elevation, sedation/analgesia, hyperosmolar therapy, mild hyperventilation, and ventricular drainage.
- Late-tier therapies for ICP management include decompressive craniectomy, continuous paralytic administration, and barbiturate coma.
- EVD placement allows for simultaneous ICP monitoring and CSF drainage.
- Surgical evacuation of mass lesions can help alleviate the ICP elevation. It can be followed by replacement of the bone flap (craniotomy) or removal of the flap (primary decompressive craniectomy).
- Decompressive craniectomy is considered when ICP levels are greater than 25 mm Hg for more than 1–12 h.
- Cranioplasty is usually performed weeks to months after the TBI to allow for recovery.

Questions

1. When should decompressive craniectomy be considered for TBI patients?
2. What is the difference between primary and secondary craniectomy?
3. What are the common complications of decompressive craniectomy?
4. When should cranioplasty be performed?

Pivot Points

- Studies have shown a positive relationship between the size of craniectomy and reduction of ICP level; the larger the craniectomy, the better the ICP control. However, larger craniectomies were also found to be associated with increased likelihood of development of posttraumatic hydrocephalus.
- If it is anticipated that a patient might need to eventually undergo right craniectomy due to right-sided mass lesion and/or right-to-left brain swelling and midline shift, then the ICP monitor can be initially placed in the left frontal region. This can spare the patient another procedure after the craniectomy to move the ICP monitor from the right frontal site.
- It is important to adequately counsel the patient's family about expectations of craniectomy. Literature has shown that although decompressive craniectomy can reduce mortality, it was also associated with higher rates of patients with vegetative states or significant disabilities or dependence.

Oral Boards Review: Complications Pearls

- TBI and subsequent decompressive craniectomy can be complicated by post-traumatic hydrocephalus, subdural hygroma, or syndrome of the trephined. The latter can be reversed by cranioplasty.
- The most common complication of cranioplasty is infection.

Further Reading

American College of Surgeons. Trauma Quality Improvement Program. Best practices in the management of traumatic brain injury. 2015 Jan; https://www.facs.org/~/media/files/quality%20programs/trauma/tqip/traumatic%20brain%20injury%20guidelines.ashx

Carney N, Totten AM, O'Reilly C, et al. Guidelines for the management of severe traumatic brain injury, Fourth Edition. *Neurosurgery*. 2017 Jan 1;80(1):6–15. https://www.ncbi.nlm.nih.gov/pubmed/27654000

Cooper DJ, Rosenfeld JV, Murray L, et al. Decompressive craniectomy in diffuse traumatic brain injury. *N Engl J Med*. 2011 Apr 21;364(16):1493–1502. https://www.ncbi.nlm.nih.gov/pubmed/21434843

Hutchinson PJ, Kolias AG, Timofeev IS, et al. Trial of decompressive craniectomy for traumatic intracranial hypertension. *N Engl J Med*. 2016 Sep 22;375(12):1119–1130. https://www.ncbi.nlm.nih.gov/pubmed/27602507

Li LM, Timofeev I, Czosnyka M, Hutchinson PJA. The surgical approach to the management of increased intracranial pressure after traumatic brain injury. *Anesth Analg*. 2010 Sep;111(3):736–748. https://www.ncbi.nlm.nih.gov/pubmed/20686006

Acute Subdural Hematoma

*Benjamin McGahan, Nathaniel Toop, Varun Shah,
and John McGregor*

3

Case Presentation

A 45-year-old man with an unremarkable past medical history arrives to the emergency department as a level 1 trauma after being involved in an ATV accident. Per the report, the patient was not helmeted. According to reports from the scene, he was found down with eyes closed, moaning, not responsive to voice, and moved his extremities on stimulation. He was intubated in the field by EMS utilizing a combination of etomidate and succinylcholine and transported by ground to your hospital. On arrival he remains intubated and ventilated. He is bradycardic, with a heart rate of 52 and hypertensive with a blood pressure of 168/108. His hemodynamic stability is confirmed. His neurological examination is performed, and anisocoria with a 7 mm left pupil that is unreactive is noted. His right pupil is 2 mm and minimally reactive. His cough and gag are present, and his corneal reflex is intact. To noxious stimuli, he shows extensor posturing in the right upper and lower extremities. He briskly withdraws his left upper and lower extremities to noxious stimulation. His remaining physical exam is unremarkable for obvious injury.

Questions

1. What are the appropriate next studies?
2. What imaging modalities are appropriate?
3. What is the significance of the vital signs? Pupillary exam? Neurological findings on exam?
4. What diagnoses are in the differential?

Assessment and Planning

The patient has a history and physical examination findings that are concerning for acute intracranial CNS injury. The physical exam localized to the brain. The pupillary findings are concerning for a left third-nerve compression accompanying a left temporal uncal herniation associated with a left-sided acute mass lesion. The right decerebrate posturing is concerning for transtentorial herniation and midbrain compression. His vital signs of relative hypertension and bradycardia are concerning for a Cushing reflex seen in posterior fossa compression and cerebellar tonsillar herniation. Mass lesions in this setting include epidural hematoma, subdural hematoma (SDH), intracerebral hemorrhage/contusion, or some combination of them all. Other unlikely conditions could include stroke with significant edema or a postictal state.

The workup should next include serum and urine laboratory tests, including clotting studies, and emergent CT imaging. Typical advanced trauma life support evaluations and spinal injury precautions should be maintained.

Oral Boards Review: Diagnostic Pearls

- Neurological exam suggests the level and severity of injury.
- Pupillary examination suggests the laterality of the injury.
- Vital sign abnormalities can be indicative of associated hemodynamic instability in the multisystem-injured patient or brainstem compression in the comatose patient.
- Progression of neurological deficits on serial exams suggest a rapidly deteriorating condition that requires urgent evaluation and intervention.

The patient was deemed hemodynamically stable in the trauma bay, and a secondary trauma survey did not uncover obvious additional injuries. He was transported urgently for CT studies. His laboratory and coagulation studies return as his images are obtained and are normal. His images at the CT scanner reveal the findings shown in Figure 3.1.

The CT indicates an acute left SDH with mass effect and shift. There is suggestion of intraparenchymal contusion and/or subarachnoid blood in the Sylvian fissure. There is effacement of the left lateral ventricle, possible enlargement of the posterior horn of the right lateral ventricle secondary to entrapment, and significant midline shift. Acute subdural blood is hyperdense on CT. Subdural collections are crescent-shaped and cross cranial suture lines. They are more likely to be associated with intraparenchymal injury.

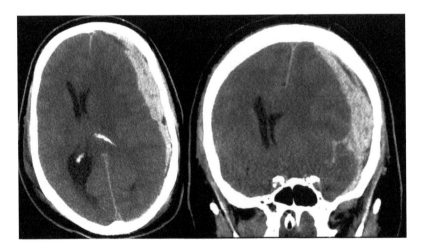

Figure 3.1 Non-contrast head CT scan, axial on the left and coronal on the right, demonstrating a hyperdense crescent shaped lesion consistent with acute blood in the subdural space. It extends across cranial sutures. There is hyperdensitiy in the left Sylvian fissure. There is significant mass effect with compression of the left lateral ventricle and midline shift to the right.

The most common inciting factor for the development of a SDH is cranial trauma resulting in translational or rotational movement of the brain parenchyma in relation to the fixed calvarium, dural sinuses, and draining veins. This causes shearing of these bridging veins that drain the cortex into a cerebral venous sinus. The high association with parenchyma injury means that cortical surface vascular injury may also result in SDH and that traumatic neurological injury is more likely. While low-pressure venous bleeds are the most common sources of subdurals, the association with cortical injury allows for arterial causes as well. Spontaneous bleeds can also occur, often in settings including coagulopathy, sickle cell disease, thrombocytopenia, cerebral atrophy, and CSF leak, among others. Acute SDHs can also be encountered following external ventricular drain or ventricular shunt placement.

Depending on the cause and the findings on CT and physical exam, patients with an acute SDH can exhibit a wide spectrum of clinical consequence, from remaining asymptomatic to progressive brain herniation and death. Regardless of the etiology, the potential for neurological injury demands that any suspicion for SDH undergo urgent evaluation. The acuity of any suspected intracranial bleed is most accurately assessed using two modalities repeated over time: physical examination and radiographic studies.

Neurological examination findings have utility in the evaluation of an acute SDH, and progression of deficits suggest intervention. The neurosurgeon's examination should focus on readily obtainable objective measurements of consciousness. The Glasgow Coma Scale (GCS) is an extensively evaluated, widely accepted, and easily repeatable/transferable examination tool for such patients (Table 3.1).

A patient's best scores in each of these three components is added together, allowing for a range of scores from 3 (deep comatose state) to 15 (normal exam). A GCS of 8 or less is generally defined as comatose.

An additional important aspect of the neurological exam in such patients is the pupillary exam. A patient's pupils can reveal important minute-to-minute intracranial changes in intracranial pressure (ICP) or size of mass lesions in a trauma patient, including progression to uncal herniation. Furthermore, a pupillary exam may be the only readily obtainable neurological assessment in a recently intubated patient who has been pharmacologically paralyzed. Important findings include unequal pupils, nonreactive pupils, and the ominous unilateral or bilateral large and nonresponsive pupil. The dilated

Table 3.1
Glasgow Coma Scale

Best motor response	Best verbal response	Best ocular response
1: No motor response	1: No verbal response (including intubation)	1: No ocular response
2: Decerebrate posturing	2: Incomprehensible sounds	2: Opens eyes to pain
3: Decorticate posturing	3: Inappropriate words	3: Opens eyes to voice
4: Withdrawal	4: Confused	4: Opens eyes spontaneously
5: Localization	5: Fully oriented	
6: Following commands		

pupil is also suggestive of the most likely side of a mass lesion, either hemorrhage, edema, or tumor. Vital signs abnormalities such as relative hypertension and bradycardia in the comatose patient can be indicative of the Cushing's reflex that is associated with brainstem compression at the cervico-medullary junction and cerebellar tonsillar herniation. Patients who have abnormal findings on these quickly ascertained measures should undergo urgent cranial imaging.

The most appropriate radiographic study in settings suggestive of intracranial hemorrhage is a head CT without contrast. This scan is usually quick to obtain and usually readily identifies acute blood products as hyperdense due to the iron-hemoglobin complexes. Typical features of acute SDHs include hyperdense crescents. These are most commonly located along either convexity but can also be found within the posterior fossa or along the tentorial or falcine dural folds. Importantly, SDHs are not confined to suture lines and can cross these to occupy an entire convexity. This feature can help differentiate SDHs from epidural hematomas. The findings of associated intraparenchymal injury and edema are more common with SDH in general than with an epidural hematoma. Size of the subdural collection and the patient's neurological exam suggest who may benefit from surgery. However, even skim subdural collections can be associated with brain shift out of proportion and neurological decline indicative of brain injury, brain edema, or ischemia and may require surgical intervention.

Questions

1. What is the significance of each of the findings on CT?
2. What aspects of history and physical exam suggest the timing for intervention for this patient?
3. How would abnormal coagulation studies affect the timing of surgery?

Decision Making

The patient has an acute SDH with mass effect, shift, parenchyma or subarachnoid injury, and a trapped and expanded contralateral ventricle. The exam suggests herniation syndromes and impending brainstem death. His neurological exam has deteriorated from the report in the field, which indicates a rapidly deteriorating condition. He requires emergent transfer to the operating room for craniotomy and evacuation of the hematoma. The surgery should not be delayed for correction of any coagulopathies. They should be corrected in an ongoing fashion intraoperatively. Any contralateral hydrocephalus should be corrected by decompression of the clot, not by preoperative interventions such as ventricular drains. Any procedures that might delay his transfer to the operating room, including ICP monitor placement or trephinations in the ER or CT should not be undertaken preoperatively.

Questions

1. What size of craniotomy should be planned?
2. Where should the incision be placed?

3. Where should the burr holes be placed?
4. What considerations for positioning of the patient for surgery are required?
5. How should the head be fixed and positioned for surgery?

Surgical Procedure

Acute SDH is a medical emergency and should be evacuated as soon as possible when the indications for surgery are met. The indications for surgery are the following:

- An SDH greater than 10 mm in thickness or midline shift of greater than 5 mm on CT scan
- An SDH of less than 10 mm in thickness and less than 5 mm midline shift and the following:
  - GCS drops by at least 2 points from time of injury to hospital admission
  - And/or asymmetric or fixed and dilated pupils
  - And/or ICP is greater than 20 mm Hg

If surgery is indicated, the patient will undergo a craniotomy as soon as possible. The *4-hour rule* is followed in patients, which states that surgery within 4 h of neurological deterioration lowers mortality.

Positioning: Most SDH patients undergoing craniotomy for convexity SDH are positioned in a supine position with the head and body turned to place the head laterally. The cervical spine will not be cleared in the comatose patient prior to surgery, so patients must be log-rolled and supported with rolls and tape to maintain spinal alignment. The head may be secured with either a Mayfield or a horseshoe headrest.

Surgery: Surgical planning in this situation should expect a large craniotomy that includes a wide decompression of the frontal, parietal, and temporal lobes. Care should be taken to avoid opening/elevating the bone overlying the venous sinuses. Anticipation of leaving the bone flap off and the dura open should be entertained. A single burr hole is unable to evacuate clotted blood by itself and should only be considered in situations in which imaging is completely unavailable and the single burr hole is an attempt to be diagnostic with plans to convert to a craniotomy afterward.

A skin incision can be either a large front-parietal-temporal question mark incision or a T-shaped trauma flap. The incision is made through the galea onto the bone. In areas with muscle, or containing the temporalis fascia, the incision is made down to the fascia, which is then split using scalpel, scissors, or cautery. Next, Raney clips or galea hemostats are applied to the scalp edges for hemostasis. Scalp retraction is accomplished using fish hooks or towel clips attached to rubber bands, which are secured to drapes, or self-retaining retractors can be used. Next, a series of burr holes are drilled; their placement depends on the size of craniotomy needed. They are placed in a paramedian location lateral to the sagittal sinus, in the pterional point, and in the low temporal fossa. Drilling ceases when dura is adequately exposed through the burr holes. The holes are widened with curettes and Kerrison punches, and dura is separated beneath the flap from the bone. The craniotomy is completed with a craniotome with a footplate or Gigli saw, and the bone flap is elevated from the dura. The dura is then incised in a manner that preserves underlying draining veins entering the sinus, either with a large fronto-parietal-temporal question mark incision or a series of radial incisions from the center of the craniotomy out to the circumference. Once the dura is dissected, irrigation and aspiration are used to evacuate the hematoma. Irrigation should be injected circumferentially into the subdural space at the bony–dural margins to facilitate further removal of blood clot. Care should be taken to minimize the chances of inducing bleeding from the sagittal sinus.

At this juncture, the decompression part of the operation is accomplished. Care can now be taken to control any bleeding at the cortical surface, scalp flap, bone margins, and dura. A small bleeding cortical surface vein or artery that is the source of the acute subdural hemorrhage can be coagulated with bipolar electrocautery as needed. Venous sinus bleeding from draining veins and the sinuses should undergo tamponade with gel foam and gentle pressure if possible. With a venous sinus injury, the possibility of air embolization and significant blood loss should be considered and discussed with the anesthesiologist. Hypotension, hypoxia, and decrease in end-tidal CO_2 should warrant action. Repositioning in Trendelenburg position, flooding the field with irrigation, and fluid resuscitation should be performed emergently. After meticulous hemostasis, attention to closure should begin. Dural tenting sutures should be placed circumferentially and lateral to the sagittal sinus to minimize postoperative epidural formation.

After decompression is performed, assessment of potential postoperative difficulties managing edema and ICP should be done. Adjuncts for management to consider include leaving the dura open with a large sheet of dural substitute over the brain, (storing the bone flap for reinsertion weeks later), evacuation of intraparenchymal hematoma, or performing a decompressive frontal or temporal lobectomy depending on underlying damage and intraoperative swelling. Consideration for placement of an ICP monitor should taken prior to completion of surgery. The patient should be sent to the ICU postoperatively.

Nonoperative management is a consideration for SDH patients with small bleeds and who are neurologically intact and remain stable. These patients need to be managed in the ICU, with ICP monitoring as indicated by the clinical condition, serial neurological observations, and repeated CT imaging to assess for any hematoma progression and to ensure neurological status does not suddenly deteriorate.

Oral Boards Review: Management Pearls

- Venous sinus injury and venous bleeding from draining veins lateral to the sinus may require special attention. Tamponade with gel foam and cottonoids should be enough. Irrigation and suctioning of midline clot should be done only with extreme caution and may not be necessary for decompression. Dural tack-up sutures should be placed along the dura just lateral to the sinus to facilitate control of sinus bleeding. Large tears in the sinus can be occluded in the anterior one-third. With posterior tears, efforts to tamponade and/or repair should be made.
- Acute SDH can rarely be associated with vascular disease or tumor. SDH in the low temporal fossa can be associated with subarachnoid hemorrhage (SAH) from a posterior communicating artery aneurysmal rupture or in the lateral Sylvian area from a middle cerebral artery aneurysmal rupture.

Convexity SDH may be associated with a cortically based arteriovenous malformation or a tumor exposed to the cortical surface.

- Traumatic acute SDH is more likely associated with cortical injury and brain edema than is epidural hematoma. If the bone cannot be replaced due to swelling, consideration for storage and delayed reinsertion should be made.
- Use of intraoperative ultrasound in the setting of an expanding or swollen hemisphere after decompression is a useful adjunct to ascertain if there is a significant intraparenchymal clot that warrants exploration and removal, or evidence of intrahemispheric blood that is expanding.

Pivot Points

- Neurological deterioration requires more rapid interventions.
- Large craniotomy flaps improve the ability to remove clot, find bleeding points for cautery, and allow for a better decompression.
- Care should be taken to avoid exposing the sagittal or transverse sinuses or tearing of the draining veins.

Aftercare

Acute SDH patients are hospitalized in the critical care unit until they are stable neurologically and medically. Vital signs; temperature; ICP monitoring; laboratory studies including complete blood counts, chemistries, and coagulation studies; and neurological examinations should be done frequently to ensure the health and recovery of the patient and to allow for a quick response to any neurological change. These patients are at risk for seizures, infections, coagulopathies, and venous thromboses in addition to neurological deterioration. Elevated ICP can be managed with hypertonic saline, mannitol, head positioning, and hyperventilation. Indications for a return to surgery include postoperative epidural hematoma, recurrence of an acute SDH, postoperative expansion of a subdural or epidural hematoma on the opposite side, expansion of an intracerebral hematoma requiring evacuation, medically refractory cerebral edema requiring craniectomy for ICP management, hydrocephalus needing temporary diversion or shunting, CSF leak, infections, or abscesses. The patient should be given perioperative antibiotics. Airway management is key in an acute SDH patient, and the intubated patient must have adequate levels of oxygenation but ventilatory pressure, volume, and shear should be minimized in an effort to preserve pulmonary function. Prolonged ventilation may require conversion of the airway to a tracheostomy.

Venous thromboembolic (VTE) complications are high in immobile patients. Acute SDH patients are frequently traumatic brain injury patients, and the VTE complication rate is 3–4 times higher in these patients than in the average neurosurgical patient. VTE prophylaxis is highly recommended in the form of mechanical prophylaxis of the lower extremities, as long as it is not contraindicated, until the patient is ambulatory. Chemical prophylaxis may be appropriate if the patient is stable and the hematoma is small and not expanding. Chemical prophylaxis is usually safe to administer 24–72 h after surgery, but some studies have shown a high hematoma recurrence rate after chemoprophylaxis. The decision to anticoagulate should ultimately be made on a case-by-case basis, and the patient's medical history and needs should be considered.

Seizure prophylaxis is another important consideration in the acute postoperative traumatic SDH patients. Seizures increase metabolic demand, in turn increasing ICP. Antiepileptic drugs decrease the rate of seizures in these patients, making them beneficial in the aftercare of acute SDH patients. Prolonged prophylaxis is not usually necessary without a documented seizure event. Nutritional management is also important in acute SDH patients. Patients in need of an enteral or parenteral feeding should be attaining full calories by postoperative day 7.

Serial imaging is a necessary part of aftercare to ensure there is no spontaneous recurrence of the hematoma. A postop imaging schedule for SDH patients is not standardized but is done early and at frequent intervals until a patient stabilizes. CT scans are indicated by assessing the patient's neurological exam and watching for any deterioration, which would prompt repeat CT. Repeat imaging and neurological status assessment will help minimize complications and ensure patients heal safely and have the best prognosis possible.

Complications and Management

Cerebral swelling can be an early complication intra- or postoperatively even with sufficient hematoma evacuation and decompression (see chapters 1 and 2 on medical and surgical management of cerebral edema). The swelling is caused by the initial injury that led to the SDH as well as the parenchymal damage. Swelling during and after acute subdural evacuation can be managed similarly to high ICPs from other pathologies: by promoting venous outflow by elevating the head of the bed, loosening cervical collars, keeping the head and neck in neutral position, hyperventilating to a $Paco_2$ of 30–35 mm Hg, increasing sedation, intravenous pain management, bonus doses of mannitol and hypertonic saline, and drainage of CSF with an external ventricular drain. In situations of intraoperative uncontrolled edema, lobectomies may need to be performed and the bone flap left off to allow closing of the scalp.

Contralateral hemorrhages, either subdural or epidural, can occur following relief of the tamponade of an acute subdural. This complication has been reported in up to 7.4% of patients and has needed additional surgery in all cases. The best strategy for management is early detection and treatment. Patients who deteriorate after decompression or who are noted to have difficulties maintaining ICP control immediately postoperatively should be considered suspicious. Early postoperative imaging and close neurological examinations are critical.

Similar to all other surgical procedures, there is risk for wound infection. Evacuation of acute subdural hemorrhages is done in an emergent fashion on wounds that are often contaminated with debris from the inciting injury. The wound infection rate is higher than in other craniotomies. Even in emergent scenarios when time is essential and circumstances less controlled, strict sterile technique is essential.

Hydrocephalus can occur following traumatic brain injury and craniotomy. The cause is controversial. Encephalomalacia from the traumatic injury could result in ventriculomegaly. Altered CSF absorption from intracranial hemorrhage can lead to a communicating hydrocephalus picture. Additionally, patients with cerebral injury are at risk for acute or delayed seizures (see Chapter 16 on seizure management).

Oral Boards Review: Complication Pearls

- Management of cerebral edema and increased ICPs does not stop after hemorrhage evacuation and craniotomy. Failure of medical management of high ICP may require CSF diversion or further surgical intervention.
- Postoperative imaging and close observation with serial neurological examinations are necessary for early identification of brain edema from contusion or stroke or of expansion of other intracranial hemorrhages including postop epidural hematoma, SDH, or intraparenchymal hematoma.
- Despite the emergent fashion of these procedures and the emphasis on speed of diagnosis, transport to the operating room, and progression to decompression in a timely manner, meticulous attention must still be paid to sterile technique and wound closure.

Evidence and Outcomes

The outcomes for acute SDH evacuation are found to be based largely on what level of preoperative neurological injury exists. The independent risk factors for poor outcome in acute SDH evacuation are increasing age, lower GCS score, and poor neurological exam. On a case-by-case basis, predicting outcomes in these patients is difficult because there are many reports of elderly patients with poor presentation who are able to make meaningful recoveries.

Further Reading

Bales JW, Bonow RH, Ellenbogen RG. Surgical management of closed head injury. In Ellenbogen RG, Sekhar LN, Kitchen N, eds. *Principles of Neurological Surgery* (4th ed.). Amsterdam: Elsevier; 2018:366–389.

Huang MC. Surgical management of traumatic brain injury. In Winn HR, ed. *Youmans and Winn Neurological Surgery* (7th ed.). Amsterdam: Elsevier; 2017:2910–2921.

Ndgir R, Yousem DM. Head trauma. In Ndgir R, Yousem DM, eds. *Neuroradiology: The Requisites* (4th ed.). Amsterdam: Elsevier; 2016:150–173.

Timmons SD. Extra-axial hematomas. In Loftus CM, ed. *Neurosurgical Emergencies*. Ebook. Stuttgart, Germany: Thieme; 2018:1–59.

Chronic Subdural Hematoma

*Nathaniel Toop, Benjamin McGahan, Varun Shah,
and John McGregor*

4

Case Presentation

An 85-year-old woman with a history of coronary artery disease, peripheral artery disease, chronic obstructive pulmonary disease (COPD), and diabetes mellitus presents to the emergency department of her own accord following a 2-week history of persistent headaches and clumsiness with her right hand. She takes daily aspirin and clopidogrel for femoral artery stents placed 3 years ago. She reports that she has had several mechanical falls recently and may have hit her head once or twice. On exam she is alert and oriented to time, place, date, and situation. Her vital signs are stable. She has no cranial nerve deficits. On motor exam, she has slight 4/5 weakness of all the muscle groups of her right upper extremity and has a positive right-sided pronator drift.

Questions

1. What are the appropriate next laboratory studies?
2. What imaging modalities are appropriate?
3. What is the significance of the history of falls? The medications? The neurological findings on exam?
4. What diagnoses are in the differential?
5. What is the timing of the workup?

Assessment and Planning

The patient's history of headache with mild right-sided weakness and right pronator drift are indicative of a left hemispheric pathology. Previous history of falls suggests the possibility of traumatic hemorrhage. The subacute nature would suggest a more chronic traumatic hemorrhage such as a chronic subdural hematoma (SDH). Other considerations include a small cortical or capsular stroke or possibly a mass lesion in the left posterior frontal lobe, such as tumor or abscess. Less likely would be some form of a postictal state following a seizure.

The workup should next include further physical exam evaluations including auscultation of heart and carotid looking for potential emboli sources; serum laboratory tests, including clotting studies; EKG looking for arrhythmia; and imaging of the brain. CT imaging is most often more efficiently obtained and can quickly evaluate for blood and mass effect. MRI is a indicated after a head CT is found to be nondiagnostic. The length of time she has had symptoms does not suggest an acute stroke event.

Oral Boards Review: Diagnostic Pearls

- Neurological exam suggests the laterality and location of the affected component of the CNS. Acute presentations of new deficits would suggest a more urgent time course and indicate the workup for a possible stroke
- Anticoagulants are risk factors for intracranial hemorrhage associated with minimal head trauma. Chronic SDH can be associated with minimal or unrecognized remote trauma. They can be spontaneous.
- Intermittent neurological deficits and/or seizures can be a consequence of cortical irritation associated with chronic hemorrhage.
- Progression of neurological deficits on serial exams suggests a rapidly deteriorating condition that requires more urgent evaluation and intervention.

The patient's laboratory studies were unremarkable. The cardiovascular evaluation including EKG was noncontributory. She was transported for CT studies of the head. Her images at the CT scanner reveals the findings shown in Figure 4.1.

The patient's imaging is consistent with a mixed acute-on-chronic SDH. There is a mixture of hypodense, isodense, and hyperdense blood overlying the left frontal lobe. There is mild left-to-right shift of the midline structures beneath the falx. There is effacement of the cortical sulci on the left.

CT imaging of acute blood shows it to be hyperdense for the first week following bleed. Subacute blood becomes isodense with brain tissue during the second week. Then, as blood becomes liquified at the chronic stage, SDHs are hypodense. Regardless of age, subdural blood can form crescents along the hemisphere, they can layer along the tentorium, or they can form in the intrahemispheric fissure. The blood is not limited at

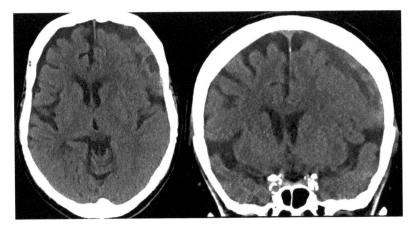

Figure 4.1 Non-contrast head CT with axial view on the left and coronal view on the right. A lesion of mixed density (hypodense, isodense and hyperdense components) is noted in the subdural space overlying the left frontal lobe. There is mass effect with mild left to right shift, and effacement of the left frontal sulci.

cranial suture lines as with an epidural hematoma. Mixed-density SDH implies multiple episodes of bleeding at different intervals into the same subdural space and that are now in various stages of degradation. Rebleeds are common into old subdural collections, and often a patient will have imaging that reveals heterogeneous densities within bleeds suggestive of bleeds that vary in age. Another important component of chronic subdural hemorrhages often seen on imaging are *septations*. Fibroblasts and fibrin formation leads to formation of membranes adjacent to liquifying blood. These can divide the subdural collections into compartments. Over time, neovascularization occurs in the membranes that can lead to multiple episodes of hemorrhage as well. The presence or absence of loculations can be an important consideration in determining a surgical approach. The majority of patient's with chronic SDHs are older than 50, and many subdurals are incurred following minor or no reported trauma. Furthermore, antiplatelet and antico-agulant medications, such as clopidogrel and aspirin, are well known to increase the risk for intracranial bleeding. Thus, this patient is a prime example of one who suffers from a chronic SDH, and her history and physical exam should prompt urgent cranial imaging.

Questions

1. What is the significance of each of the findings on CT?
2. What aspects of history and physical exam suggest the timing for intervention for this patient?
3. How would abnormal coagulation studies affect the timing of intervention?
4. What circumstances would suggest the patient would best be treated with surgery? Observation?

Decision Making

A neurosurgeon's evaluation of a patient with the preceding imaging should begin with the basics. The ABCs and Glasgow Coma Scale (GCS) score should all be assessed within the first few moments of encountering the patient. In many instances, such as the one presented here, these assessments will be unremarkable. At this point a detailed neurological exam and history should be gathered. Important features of the history include antiplatelet or anticoagulation use, recent trauma, coagulopathy history, previous diagnosis of intracranial hematoma, seizure history, and symptomatology. A physical exam should focus on deficits in strength, cranial nerves, speech, or cognition. Any neurological deficits may support surgical intervention. Patients with neurological deficits who are medically stable enough to tolerate surgery warrant intervention. Those with hemorrhages thicker than the calvarium, or hemorrhages greater than 1 cm in thickness will benefit from surgery. Bilateral subdurals should be considered for surgery earlier given the increased risk for deterioration.

Isodense subdurals can be hard to measure on head CT. CT with contrast may better outline the brain surface. Clues for mass effect can observed, including shift of midline structures, compression of the ventricles, and effacement of cortical sulci, which may indicate degree of expansion of the subdural fluid. MRI scans can often better delineate the extent and size of an isodense subdural hemorrhage. MRI takes more time to obtain than a CT.

Patients in need of surgery should have their anticoagulation reversed. This may be done emergently as surgery progresses in the deteriorating patient or over several days preoperatively in the stable patient. Patients without deficit or with a small hematoma may be observed in the hospital. Serial CT scans are needed to assess for progression of the subdural. Those that grow require evacuation. Patients who develop deficits or seizures require evacuation. Small asymptotic SDH may reabsorb with observation alone. Asymptomatic hyperdense SDH may be observed for several days then treated with evacuation as it liquifies. Hypodense hematomas that have liquified are then amenable to burr hole drainage. Mixed SDHs that have a significant hyperdense component are still clotted and require a craniotomy to evacuate.

Questions

1. What type of surgery should be planned? Bedside drain? Multiple burr holes? Or craniotomy?
2. How should the head be positioned and immobilized?
3. Where should the incision(s) and burr holes be placed?
4. What considerations for positioning of the patient for surgery are required?
5. Which burr holes should be opened first? Closed first?
6. How should multiple loculations and pial membranes be addressed at surgery?
7. When should burr hole surgery convert to craniotomy?
8. Should a drain be left postoperatively?

Surgical Procedure

Urgent hematoma evacuation is indicated in the chronic SDH patient if they have developed significant deficits, signs of herniation, or elevated ICP (i.e., asymmetric or fixed and dilated pupils) that are attributed to the chronic SDH and if these patients have a potential for recovery. Liquified subdural fluid can be evacuated through a burr hole. Burr holes need to be placed in the cranium overlying the subdural. Care should be taken not to place them over cortex because of difficulty with irrigation and increased potential for injury. The dura should be coagulated, opened in a cruciate fashion, and the edges further coagulated to prevent introduction of new blood. There is no consensus on the best way to treat chronic SDHs. One method is to irrigate through two burr holes until the saline runs clear between them. The surgeon may also use one large burr hole or small craniectomy from which to irrigate and aspirate the hematoma. Large and loculated subdurals may require multiple (three or more) burr holes in order to irrigate each cavity to remove liquified blood.

Another option is to have one burr hole with a subdural drain in place for 24–48 h. This can be performed outside of the OR. A full craniotomy for a chronic SDH is rarely required. It may be indicated in chronic SDHs that have become septated with multiple thickened membranes and unlikely to be reduced through irrigation alone. Obtaining adequate evacuation of these septated bleeds through a burr hole approach requires cautery and division of several layers of membranes, sometimes only possible via a craniotomy. Intraoperatively, conversion to a craniotomy may be required to coagulate cortical bleeders that cannot be addressed through the burr holes. Care should be taken not to strip away membranes attached to the cortical surface because of the higher risk of stroke, injury, or seizure.

Some studies have advocated for the conservative management of patients older than 70 with chronic SDHs without increased ICP, even if they have cognitive impairment that is directly attributable to the chronic SDHs. Results have shown that patients with minor head trauma were observed for 1 month, and, over the course of 4–6 weeks, their chronic SDHs disappeared or markedly reduced, and they were clinically recovered. The brain atrophy associated with old age allows for more room for subdural blood to pool without causing significant neurological dysfunction. This may be a reason that chronic SDHs may be managed nonoperatively.

Oral Boards Review: Management Pearls

- Open the upper burr hole first. This decompresses the cranium, but may keep the expanding brain away from the other burr holes until they can be opened. Close the dependent burr holes first to fill the subdural cavity with irrigation and minimize trapped air.
- Irrigate through each burr hole until the solution returns clear. A red rubber catheter may be used to irrigate into dependent spaces.
- Membranes separating loculations may need to be cauterized and divided for each chamber to be irrigated until clear. Pia surface membranes should be left intact.
- An ultrasound probe may be useful in identifying additional loculations.
- Leaving a postoperative drain has been advocated to reduce the incidence of recurrent SDH.
- Asymptomatic initial and residual subdural collections can be successfully managed nonoperatively with serial CT scans to follow the resolution of the fluid.

Pivot Points

- Surgery is indicated for patients with symptoms of cortical irritation or mass effect who can tolerate and will benefit from the surgery.
- Decompression and irrigation of inflammatory old blood products are the main goals. Complete return of the brain to normal position is not commonly seen intraoperatively.
- Uncontrolled hemorrhage may require conversion to a craniotomy.
- Avoid taking down the membranes adherent to the cortical pial surface and avoid venous sinuses or their draining veins.

Aftercare

Postoperatively, these patients need to be monitored in the ICU. Vital signs; temperature; ICP monitoring; laboratory studies including complete blood counts, chemistries, and coagulation studies; and neurological examinations should be done frequently to ensure the health and recovery of the patient and to allow for a quick response to any neurological change. These patients are at risk for seizures, infections, coagulopathies, and venous thromboses in addition to neurological deterioration. If the patient has a subdural drain in place, prophylactic antibiotics should be administered until the removal of the drain.

Venous thromboembolic (VTE) complications are high in immobile patients. VTE prophylaxis in the form of mechanical prophylaxis of the lower extremities is highly recommended as long as it is not contraindicated, until the patient is ambulatory. Chemical prophylaxis may be appropriate if the patient is stable and the hematoma is resolved or any residual is small and not expanding. Chemical prophylaxis is usually safe to administer 24–72 h after surgery, but some studies have shown a high hematoma recurrence rate after chemoprophylaxis. The decision to anticoagulate should ultimately be made on a case-by-case basis, and the patient's medical history and needs should be considered.

In the nonoperative patient ICP, neurological function, and imaging should be assessed repeatedly to ensure that the patient is not deteriorating. Seizure prophylaxis is required in patients who present with or develop seizures. Prolonged prophylaxis is not usually necessary without a documented seizure event. Nutritional optimization is important in these patients.

Serial imaging is a necessary part of aftercare to ensure there is no spontaneous recurrence of the hematoma. Postoperative imaging for SDH patients is variable, but is done early in the postoperative period, repeated as necessary, and again in intervals after discharge until subdural fluid resolves. In the early postoperative period and beyond, a deteriorating neurological exam should prompt repeat CT. Repeat imaging and neurological status assessment will ensure patients heal safely and have the best prognosis possible. Maximizing these postoperative outcomes will improve the morbidity and mortality of the chronic SDH patient.

Complications and Management

Postoperative mortality for evacuation of chronic SDHs has been found to be around 2–5%. Mortality has been related to age and clinical status at presentation, medical comorbidities, and coagulopathies.

The rate of postoperative recurrence of chronic SDH is approximately 10–20%. Associative factors with recurrence are bilateral subdural bleeds, perioperative anticoagulants or antiplatelet agents, and intracranial air. Postop subdural drains may reduce the risk. Patients with fluid collections following evacuation do not necessarily need to be taken back to surgery for reoperation. Radiographic fluid collections are common: it has been found that only 20% of a chronic SDH needs to be removed to alleviate higher ICP and provide symptom relief. The need for reoperation is based on clinical deterioration and worsened midline shift or finding of an acute postop hematoma that is larger than that at preop.

Other complications include focal brain injury, seizures, tension pneumocephalus, and empyema. Known surgical risks are surgical site infections, hospital-acquired infections, thromboembolism, and myocardial infarcts. Because chronic SDHs are frequently found in the elderly, many of these known surgical risks have a higher prevalence and/or greater morbidity than comparable operations in younger, healthier patients undergoing surgery. All attempts should be made to optimize the patient prior to surgery and after surgery to prevent these known surgical risks.

Oral Boards Review: Complication Pearls

- Care should be taken to place burr holes over subdural collections and not cortex. Image guidance and intraoperative ultrasound may be useful adjuncts to prevent cortical injury.
- Minimization of postoperative intracranial air is important and can be accomplished with proper positioning, proper placement of burr holes, adequate irrigation, and consideration of the order of burr hole closure.
- Postoperative imaging and close observation with serial neurological examinations are necessary for early identification of new or recurrent hemorrhage.
- Meticulous attention must still be paid to sterile technique and wound closure.

Evidence and Outcomes

As the population ages, chronic SDH becomes more prevalent in neurosurgical practice. The current standard understanding is that surgical management is the best treatment for symptomatic chronic SDHs. Evidence is accumulating that may shift more patients to observation status. Further research is needed into the best surgical techniques and the role of medical management.

Further Reading

Bales JW, Bonow RH, Ellenbogen RG. Surgical management of closed head injury. In Ellenbogen RG, Sekhar LN, Kitchen N, eds. *Principles of Neurological Surgery* (4th ed.). Amsterdam: Elsevier; 2018:366–389.

Huang MC. Surgical management of traumatic brain injury. In Winn HR, ed. *Youmans and Winn Neurological Surgery* (7th ed.). Amsterdam: Elsevier; 2017:2910–2921.

Ndgir R, Yousem DM. Head trauma. In Ndgir R, Yousem DM, eds. *Neuroradiology: The Requisites* (4th ed.). Amsterdam: Elsevier; 2016:150–173.

Timmons SD. Extra-axial hematomas. In Loftus CM, ed. *Neurosurgical Emergencies*. Ebook. Stuttgart, Germany: Thieme; 2018:1–59.

Epidural Hematoma

Lydia Kaoutzani and Martina Stippler

5

A 38-year-old bicyclist fell going downhill in steep terrain. He was confused at the scene, but the confusion cleared. However, a friend urged him to go to the emergency department (ED) to be checked out. In the ED, he becomes drowsy. On examination, the patient now has a Glasgow Coma Scale (GCS) score of 7. He only moves his left side, his pupils are equal and reactive, and his brainstem reflexes are intact.

Questions

1. What should be the next step in this patient's care?
2. What criteria determine whether a patient presenting with trauma should undergo a head CT scan as part of the initial evaluation?
3. What is the differential diagnosis in the setting of head trauma in this patient?

Assessment and Planning

As in any trauma case, the first step in this patient's care is to maintain airway and circulation. If his GCS has deteriorated to 7, he will need to be intubated first to secure his airway. He also now has a fixed neurological deficit that is lateralizing to the left side. Therefore, a head CT scan is warranted. A significant proportion of patients presenting with epidural hematomas (EDH) have the classically described lucid interval. This is a period right after the head injury when the patient has full consciousness, after which the patient falls into coma. It is important not to miss this interval in a patient who presents to the ED during the awake period. Others patients present with signs and symptoms that indicate elevated intracranial pressure (ICP). About 20–50% of patients with an EDH are comatose when they arrive in the ED or directly before surgery. This further warrants a head CT scan.

A fundamental breakthrough for the diagnosis of all brain traumatic injuries was the advent of CT. In this case the patient presented after his lucid interval, and it is clear he needs imaging. It is more challenging to know which patient presenting after minor trauma should have a head CT scan. There are two externally validated rules regarding when to require a CT scan after mild traumatic brain injury (TBI). One is the Canadian CT Head Rule (CCTHR); the other is the New Orleans Criteria (NOC). These rules have 100% sensitivity for neurosurgical lesions and 83–98% sensitivity for nonoperative lesions. Neither rule addresses the presence of coagulopathy and anticoagulation, which others deem important risk factors for intracranial bleeding. These criteria were updated

Table 5.1
Factors to consider when determining need of CT in patients with head injury

Indications for urgent CT scan:	Indications for lower threshold for CT scan:
• Evidence of skull fracture—basal, depressed, or open	• Age >60 y
	• Persistent anterograde amnesia
• Abnormal results of neurological examination	• Retrograde amnesia >30 min
• Seizure	• Coagulopathy
• Vomiting >1 time	• Fall from >5 stairs or >3 feet
• High-risk mechanism (e.g., ejection from vehicle; pedestrian or cyclist vs. automobile)	• Intoxication (examination unreliable)
	• LOC >30 min
• Decreasing GCS score or persistently decreased GCS score of <15	• Mechanism and location of injury
	• Social factors (e.g., abusive situation at home, language barriers preclude accurate history)

CT, computed tomography; GCS, Glasgow Coma Scale; LOC, loss of consciousness.

in 2007, and several factors were identified as indicators for urgent CT scanning of the head after trauma (Table 5.1).

The classic CT scan finding for EDH is that of a lens-like (biconvex) shape. This is the result of the arterial bleeding that causes the detachment of the dura mater from the inner surface of the skull. The bleeding is from the bone rupturing an interosseous artery or venous sinus. Venous EDHs can cross the midline and are often found under the transverse or sagittal sinus. However, one should remember that only 84% of EDHs present with the classic biconvex shape on CT images. The remaining cases (16%) present with the side against the skull appearing convex and the side along the brain being straight.

A small but still important subgroup of patients are those presenting with a posterior fossa EDH. These patients usually have no symptoms, but they deteriorate suddenly from developing pressure on the brainstem.

Delayed EDH is also a phenomenon that must be considered in patients who suddenly deteriorate after trauma and a negative head CT scan. It is seen in patients in whom the first CT was obtained less than 6 h following injury. The initial CT scan in these patients has been obtained "too soon," and the EDH did not have time to develop or is very small and missed. That is also why many patients with a history of TBI are observed before being discharged.

The differential diagnosis for this patient is an intracranial hemorrhage. Skull fracture on the CT scan and the lucid interval make an EDH more likely, but any intracranial mass lesion could present this way. He also could have a posttraumatic seizure and now is presenting with Todd's paralysis.

A CT scan (Figures 5.1 and 5.2) was obtained within 2 h of the injury and showed a left-sided skull fracture and convex extra-axial hematoma consistent with an EDH with midline shift.

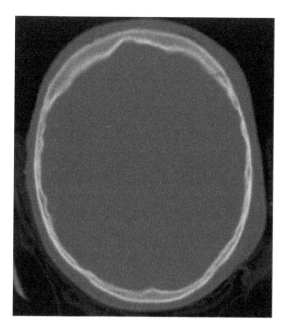

Figure 5.1 This is a head CT depicts an acute arterial right sided epidural hematoma. Please note the typical convex shape typical for a epidural hematoma.

Although EDHs are not the most frequently seen intracranial injury in trauma, they present an emergency situation that can result in significant mortality if not diagnosed and treated in a timely manner. The incidence of surgical and nonsurgical EDH among TBI patients ranges from 2.7% to 4%. A patient in a coma has a higher likelihood (about

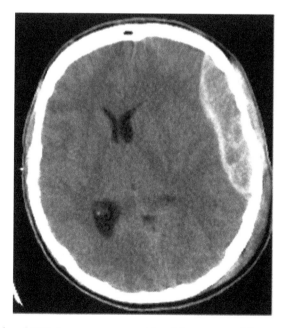

Figure 5.2 This head CT shows a venus epidural hematoma. The proximity to the sagittal venus sinus and the fact the hematoma is almost crossing the midline should raise the suspicion of this epidural hematoma originating from venous sinus injury.

9%) of harboring an EDH. In most patients who present in a coma, the EDH is operative. The peak incidence of EDH is from 20 to 30 years of age. Because of the young age of the high-risk group, EDH contributes to a significant public health burden. EDH also are seen in children from 6 to 10 years old. Traffic-related accidents, falls, and assaults account for about half (53%) of all EDH.

An EDH has been described as the accumulation of blood in a "potential" space, which is that of the outer layer of the dura mater and the skull. Bleeding is usually the result of traumatic rupture of the middle meningeal artery, which is the largest branch of the external carotid artery and the largest of the meningeal vessels. The tear usually occurs secondary to temporal bone fracture. Various series involving both adult and pediatric patients found that arterial bleeding was responsible for the formation of an EDH in one-third of the adult patients, while this percentage was significantly smaller in the pediatric population.

Approximately one-third to one-half of all patients with EDHs have other associated findings such as skull fractures, subdural hematoma (SDH), and/or intraparenchymal hemorrhage (IPH). These associated lesions, especially brain injury, are related to worse patient outcomes.

Various authors have examined the prevalence and impact of skull fractures on EDHs. A study found that up to 87% of linear skull fractures are associated with an extradural hematoma. Others studied the functional outcome of 200 patients who underwent surgery for EDHs but did not find an association between unfavorable functional outcome and cranial fractures. Others report that the presence of a fracture overlying a major vessel or major sinus in a patient with a small EDH makes a surgical intervention more likely.

Bleeding due to traumatic rupture of venous sinuses can also occur. The onset of neurological deterioration is less acute with a venous hemorrhage than an arterial one, but the lacerated sinus adds a challenge to any operative intervention. In patients with depressed skull fractures overlying the sagittal or transverse sinus, the EDH should be considered venous (Figure 5.3). A vertex EDH or an EDH that crosses the midline should raise the suspicion of this being a venous EDH from a sinus laceration.

A CT angiogram/venogram can help clarify the relationship of the venous sinus to the EDH and should be considered if it can be obtained with minimal or no delay of the operative intervention.

Oral Boards Review: Diagnostic Pearls

- Don't miss an EDH if the patient presents in the lucid interval.
- Be aware of delayed EDHs if the first CT scan was obtained less than 6 h following the injury.
- Differentiate between an arterial and a venous EDH.

This patient has a symptomatic EDH larger than 30 cc, which is an indication for surgery according to surgical guidelines. This patient should be taken immediately to the operating room for an emergency craniotomy for EDH evacuation and be given 0.7 g /kg of mannitol on the way to the OR.

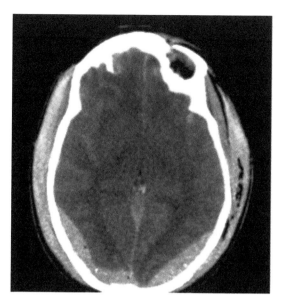

Figure 5.3 This the same CT scan as Fig 5.1 shows in a bone window highlighting the left frontal linear skull fracture causing the underlaying epidural hematoma.

Questions

1. What is the most likely cause of this bleeding?
2. When do you suspect a venous EDH?
3. What is your next step in management of this patient?

Decision Making

The current school of thought is that patients who present with a small (≤10 mm maximal thickness) EDH with no neurological symptoms can be treated conservatively. Patients with no focal neurological deficits and a GCS of greater than 8 with an EDH volume of less than 30 cc, a midline shift of less than 5 mm, and an EDH thickness of less than 15 mm also can be managed nonoperatively.

What seems to be important in this setting, however, is the need for continuous monitoring of the patient's neurological status, as well as initial short-term follow-up with a head CT scan if the patient is managed nonoperatively. Coordination between different physician teams caring for the patient and a nursing staff well-versed in neurological examination is paramount when caring for TBI patients, especially patients with EDH.

On the other hand, even patients neurologically intact with a normal GCS but an EDH of greater than 30 cc should undergo surgery because of the high risk of sudden deterioration. Also, a midline shift of greater than 5 mm and an EDH thickness of greater than 15 mm, even in the setting of a GCS score of 14–15, are indications for surgery (Table 5.2).

Whenever possible, the cause of the EDH should be identified preoperatively when considering surgery so the craniotomy can be centered over the possible bleeding source. If this is not possible, or the bleeding source is uncertain, then a standard

Table 5.2
Indications for operative versus nonoperative treatment in epidural hematoma (EDH)

Criteria for surgical treatment		Criteria for nonsurgical treatment	
GCS 3–15 GCS 14–15	• Volume >30 cc • Midline shift >5 mm • Thickness >15 mm	No focal neurological deficits & GCS >8	• EDH volume <30 cc • Midline shift <5 mm • Thickness <15 mm

GCS, Glasgow Coma Scale.

frontotemporal-parietal trauma craniotomy should be considered, which gives enough room to identify the bleeding source. If the bleeding source can be identified preoperatively, a more localized craniotomy can be considered. Some authors recommend opening the dura in all cases to rule out an underlying SDH. The dura definitely should be opened if the brain still looks full after the EDH has been removed. Also, if there is preoperative suspicion of an SDH, or if no EDH is found, the dura should be opened. Circumferential tack-up stitches and a central tack-up stitch, which is placed when the bone flap is replaced, are paramount to reducing postoperative recurrence of EDH.

Preoperative suspicion and a combination of surgical techniques are important for venous sinus injury management in trauma. In some cases, a craniotomy extending to either side of midline might be appropriate to deal with the sinus injury under direct vision. Others prefer a craniotomy leaving a strip of bone in midline over the lacerated sinus area so that bilateral tack-up or hitch stitches can control the bleeding from the sinus. Direct suture repair of the venous sinus can be augmented with a muscle patch if the dura cannot be completely approximated.

Questions

1. What are the criteria for nonoperative management of an EDH?
2. How do you lower the chances of recurrence of EDH postoperatively?
3. How do you handle and prevent massive bleeding from a lacerated sinus intraoperatively?

Surgical Procedure

When originally described, EDHs were reported to have mortality rates greater than 80%. Today, with prompt diagnosis and treatment, the mortality rate of EDHs has declined.

The surgery of choice for an EDH is craniotomy because the goal is to evacuate the hematoma and relieve the ICP. The planned craniotomy can be a large frontotemporal-parietal craniotomy or a more localized craniotomy over the EDH. If a venous EDH from a lacerated venous sinus is suspected, the craniotomy should be planned accordingly to allow access to and control of the sinus. Planning a craniotomy on either side of the lacerated sinus, but leaving a strip of bone over the lacerated sinus area, might allow for access and control at the same time.

Craniotomy also is pertinent if a small localized craniotomy is performed, to plan ahead and allow conversion to 11 × 14 cm craniectomy if brain swelling is encountered.

The interval between injury and definitive surgical treatment is especially important. Patients with anisocoria who had surgery within 70 min have had favorable outcomes. Moreover, patients treated within 2 h did better compared to patients who were operated on in a more delayed fashion. There is evidence that a delay between initial presentation and surgical evacuation contributes to poorer patient outcomes, and this is the reason for the ongoing debate about whether it is optimal for patients to undergo surgical treatment at the nearest hospital or at a more specialized center.

Oral Boards Review: Management Pearls

- Know the criteria of operative and nonoperative management of EDH (Table 5.2).
- If you suspect a venous EDH from a venous sinus injury, be prepared to treat the injured sinus and other complications that can arise from it (air embolus, massive blood loss).
- Place tack-up suture circumferentially and in the center of your bone flap.

Pivot Points

- If a depressed skull fracture overlies a venous sinus, get a CT angiogram to evaluate for venous sinus thrombosis.
- If the brain still looks full after EDH evacuation, open the dura and look to rule out a subdural component.
- If the patient has a GCS of 8 or lower, place multimodality monitors or ICP monitor.

Aftercare

Most patients with EDH have minimal to no underlying brain injury and, even with a poor neurological examination preoperatively, most patients emerge from the coma postoperatively. Therefore, patients should be given a chance to wake up before placing intracranial monitors. If the patient has not awakened after adequate time to wean off the anesthesia, a postoperative CT should be obtained to evaluate for recurrent EDH or other intracranial pathology. If no mass lesion can be found and the GCS is less than 8 without following commands, intracranial multimodality monitoring should be placed. If a severe TBI is present, the severe TBI protocol should be followed and coordinated with other care necessary for systemic injuries.

Complications and Management

Thorough operative planning can help to manage venous sinus bleeding intraoperatively if a venous EDH is suspected. In addition, an adequately large craniotomy will help to achieve adequate hemostasis to prevent postoperative reaccumulation of the EDH. Epidural drain placement and tack-up sutures can mitigate this as well.

It is important to keep an open mind regarding how severe the underlying brain injury will be. Most EDH have minimal parenchymal injury, but if the patient presents with a poor neurological examination, it can be difficult to tell preoperatively. Be prepared to convert to a hemicraniectomy if the dura is tense and the brain is swollen. If a localized craniotomy was performed, make sure you have room to increase the craniotomy and incision to have a craniotomy at least 11 × 14 cm in size.

Oral Boards Review: Complications Pearls

- Make your craniotomy large enough so you can find the source of the bleeding.
- Be prepared to perform an 11 × 14 cm hemicraniectomy if the brain is swollen.
- If the patient does not wake up to a GCS of at least 9, consider multimodality intracranial monitoring.

Evidence and Outcomes

The mortality in patients in all age groups and GCS scores undergoing surgery for evacuation of EDH is approximately 10%. The mortality in comparable pediatric case series is approximately 5%. This is a much lower mortality than is seen in other operative TBIs. By comparison, the mortality for SDH is 30–50% and about 30% in severe TBI. The reason for this difference is the degree of underlying brain injury. In EDH, most of the decreased level of consciousness is thought to be more from increased ICP from the mass effect of the EDH and less from underlying injury to the brain parenchyma. SDHs are associated with a much higher degree of underlying brain injury, hence their outcome is significantly worse when compared to EDH.

Even a patient with a poor neurological exam can have a good outcome if the EDH is evacuated within 2–4 h of deterioration. Table 5.3 lists factors contributing to the outcome from EDH.

Table 5.3
Factors determining outcome from epidural hematoma

Glasgow Coma Scale
Age
Pupillary abnormalities
Associated intracranial lesions
Time between neurological deterioration and surgery
Intracranial pressure

Further Reading

Behera SK, Senapati SB, Mishra SS, Das S. Management of superior sagittal sinus injury encountered in traumatic head injury patients: Analysis of 15 cases. *Asian J Neurosurg.* 2015;10(1):17–20. doi: 10.4103/1793-5482.151503. https://www.ncbi.nlm.nih.gov/pubmed/?term=behera+superior+sagittal+sinus+injury

Bor-Seng-Shu E, Aguiar PH, de Almeida Leme RJ, Mandel M, Andrade AF, Marino R Jr. Epidural hematomas of the posterior cranial fossa. *Neurosurg Focus.* 2004;16 (2): ECP1, Clinical Pearl 1, 2004. https://www.ncbi.nlm.nih.gov/pubmed/?term=edson+epidural+heamotaomas+of+the+posterior+cranical+fossa

Bullock MR, Chesnit R, Ghajar J, et al. Surgical management of acute epidural hematomas. *Neurosurgery.* 2006;58(suppl 3): S7–S15; discussion Si-iv

Haydel MJ, Preston CA, Mills TJ, Luber S, Blaudeau E, DeBlieux PM. Indications for computed tomography in patients with minor head injury. *N Engl J Med.* 2000;343(2):100–105.

Langlois JA, Rutland-Brown W, Wald MM. The epidemiology and impact of traumatic brain injury: a brief overview. *J Head Trauma Rehabil.* 2006;21(5):375–378. https://www.ncbi.nlm.nih.gov/pubmed/16983222

Stiell IG, Wells GA, Vandemheem K, et al. The Canadian CT head rule for patients with minor head injury. *Lancet.* 2001; 357(9266):1391–1396. https://www.ncbi.nlm.nih.gov/pubmed/11356436

Injury to the Dural Venous Sinuses

Tarek Y. El Ahmadieh, Christopher J. Madden,
and Shelly D. Timmons

6

Case Presentation

A 46-year-old woman presented to the emergency department (ED) after a fall from height during which she struck her head. Her past medical history was significant for drug abuse and bipolar disorder. On arrival, she was noted to be alert to person and city but not to situation or date. Her speech was slow and slurred. Her facial motor examination was symmetric, and the eye exam showed reactive symmetrical pupils and intact extraocular muscle movements. She followed commands in all four extremities with normal strength and sensory function. She had no pronator drift. Her Glasgow Coma Scale (GCS) score was 14. She complained of a severe headache.

Questions

1. What are the appropriate next steps?
2. What imaging modalities should be considered?

Assessment and Planning

As the patient had fallen from a significant height, she underwent a full trauma evaluation using standard advanced trauma life support (ATLS) protocols. Because of the mechanism of injury, complaint of headache, and the abnormal neurological exam, a head CT is an appropriate next step. A spine CT was also ordered given the mechanism of injury and spine tenderness to percussion. The patient did not have any other injuries noted on the trauma survey. The spine CT showed no evidence of fracture or dislocation, but the head CT revealed a left occipital nondepressed skull fracture (Figure 6.1A,B,C) with an underlying 3 × 9 cm hematoma in the left occipital region with extension to the posterior cranial fossa (Figure 6.2A,B). The likely diagnosis was epidural hematoma (EDH) secondary to venous sinus injury given the location over the left transverse sinus. Standard trauma labs were drawn and the patient was type and screened for blood. The neurosurgery team was consulted emergently.

EDH most commonly occurs as a result of injury to the middle meningeal artery or its branches, resulting in a temporal fossa EDH and sometimes herniation from rapid expansion and mass effect on the temporal lobe with compression of the brainstem. Other causes of EDH include injury to the middle meningeal vein, the diploic veins of bone, or the dural venous sinuses. EDH of the occipital/suboccipital area is

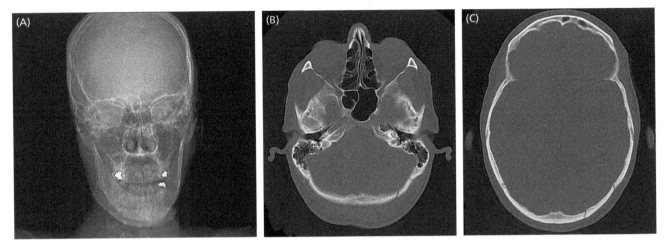

Figure 6.1 (A) Anteroposterior plain skull film. (B,C) Axial CT brain showing left occipital skull fracture extending down to suboccipital bone.

less common. In cases where it is present, the venous sinus is the source of epidural bleeding in as many as 32–42% of cases. A noncontrasted plain CT scan of the brain is considered the most appropriate initial imaging modality to assess these lesions in the ED. A characteristic finding would be a hyperdense, extracerebral biconvex lesion that does not cross dural attachments. There is no strong evidence in the literature that supports a role for vascular imaging (such as CT or MRI venograms) in the acute setting, though these may help localize an injury and may be obtained if time allows. In many cases, surgery should not be delayed for vascular imaging as the decision making is dictated by the patient's often rapidly deteriorating neurological exam. Decisions are made based on the lesion size and location, clinical presentation (including pupil examination and GCS score), and risks and benefits of the procedure considering the overall systemic traumatic injury burden.

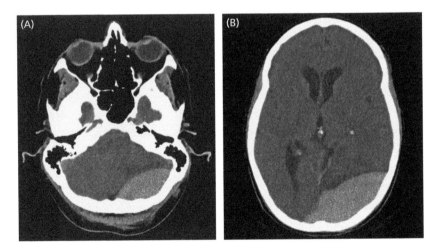

Figure 6.2 (A,B) Axial CT brain showing large left occipital/suboccipital epidural hematoma with mass effect.

Oral Boards Review: Diagnostic Pearls

- CT head is the modality of choice to screen for traumatic brain injury in the trauma patient.
- EDH in the occipital/suboccipital region (or at the vertex) should raise concern for venous sinus injury especially (though not exclusively) with depressed fractures.
- CT or MRI venograms may document a site of venous bleeding, although this is of questionable value in surgical planning.

Questions

1. Is the patient appropriate for observation given the current neurological exam, or is this a surgical lesion that requires emergent evacuation?
2. If surgery is considered, are there any special preoperative considerations?
3. Is the bleeding arterial or venous, and does that affect decision making?

Decision Making

In this case, though the patient had relatively mild neurological symptoms, the decision was made to take the patient to the operating room because of the large hematoma size, its extension to the posterior cranial fossa, and the associated mass effect. Evidence-based guidelines on the surgical management of cranial trauma state that an acute EDH with a volume greater than 30 cm³ should be evacuated surgically irrespective of the GCS score. Further recommendations state that EDHs of any volume associated with anisocoria in a patient with GCS 3–8 (i.e., in coma) be evacuated urgently. Expectant management with serial CT scans and frequent neurological checks can be considered in an EDH with *all* of the following characteristics: volume less than 30 cm³, thickness less than 1.5 cm, midline shift less than 5 mm, GCS score greater than 8, *and* absence of focal neurological deficits. However, these guidelines may not apply in the posterior fossa. Symptomatic hematomas usually warrant surgical treatment as do those that progress in size or are associated with neurological deterioration.

EDH of the posterior fossa typically has a lower threshold for surgical evacuation, given the smaller size of the posterior compartment and risk of compression of the brainstem. According to the same evidence-based guidelines, posterior fossa lesions should be surgically evacuated if they are associated with *any* of the following: mass effect from the hematoma, neurological dysfunction, or deterioration referable to the lesion. Mass effect is evidenced by distortion, dislocation, or obliteration of the fourth ventricle; compression or obliteration of the basal cisterns; or obstructive hydrocephalus.

In the case of suspected venous sinus injury, an EDH that does not meet size criteria for evacuation and is felt to be of venous origin (presumably lower pressure) may be observed carefully with frequent repeat head CTs in a hospital with adequate neurocritical care nursing available, as well as ready availability of a neurosurgeon on call to that institution and immediate access to an OR. This is because a deterioration in the neurological examination or an expanding hematoma may require emergent surgical evacuation.

EDH resulting from injury to a dural venous sinus is reportedly associated with a higher mortality rate as compared to EDH of arterial origin. This has been attributed to an overall larger hematoma size and lower GCS score upon initial presentation. Hematoma extension to the posterior fossa, as seen in this case, can increase the mortality rate significantly by brainstem compression. Dural venous sinus injury is often associated with depressed skull fractures and usually occurs as a result of more severe trauma (as compared to EDH of other etiologies); thus there is a higher probability of both other brain injury (such as diffuse axonal injury) and other systemic injuries. When possible, these lesions can be managed conservatively if the hematoma is not causing significant mass effect and the patient is neurologically intact. This may sometimes be a reasonable approach to avoid the possibility of massive bleeding during attempts to elevate a depressed skull fracture near the sinus.

EDH resulting from dural venous sinus injury is also associated with a higher rate of intra- and postoperative morbidity and a lower rate of favorable outcome as compared to EDH of other etiology. Controlling bleeding from a venous sinus laceration can be challenging and is often associated with significant blood loss. As part of preoperative trauma workup, a complete blood count (including red blood cell count, hemoglobin, hematocrit, and platelet count), as well as coagulation parameters should be tested and a history of any previous antiplatelet or anticoagulant use should be obtained (if possible). Reversing the effect of antithrombotic medications in a timely fashion can reduce the risk of hematoma progression and improve intraoperative bleeding control. In addition, it is very important to obtain a type and crossmatch for blood products (packed red blood cells, fresh frozen plasma, platelets, or whole blood) as part of preoperative workup in order to have them immediately available for intraoperative use.

Questions

1. What is the timing for intervention in this patient?
2. What would be an appropriate surgical positioning and approach?
3. In addition to concern for bleeding, is there another intraoperative concern associated with this procedure?

Surgical Procedure

The patient was taken to the operating room immediately because of the large size of the hematoma and because of concern that progression of the posterior fossa component would cause brainstem compression. In a patient with neurological decline and imminent herniation (e.g., a coma patient with anisocoria), immediate surgical decompression is indicated. In cases where the patient is not as neurologically compromised, preoperative assessment of the risk factors associated with each EDH can be undertaken, but because of the risk of expansion and further neurological decline, if the decision is made to proceed to surgery it should be undertaken expeditiously. The guidelines report insufficient data to support one surgical treatment approach over another, but the body of the literature favors a craniotomy or craniectomy (over burr holes) for complete hematoma evacuation and potential identification of the bleeding source.

After induction of general anesthesia and intubation, the patient was placed in the prone position on gel rolls with the head secured in a Mayfield. The occipital/suboccipital area was prepped and draped in normal sterile fashion. A long left paramedian incision was made extending down to the level of C2. A Bovie monopolar cautery and subperiosteal sharp dissection was used to expose the bone of both occipital and suboccipital regions on the left side. Self-retaining retractors were then placed. A large fracture extending from the occipital bone to the subocciput near the mastoid was noted. Burr holes were placed in the occipital region and suboccipitally. Hematoma was encountered under the burr holes in both regions and evacuated using suction. The drill with a footplate was then used to remove two separate bones flaps: one in the posterior fossa and another in the occipital region, leaving a strip of bone overlying the sinus. The dura and the sinus had been stripped away from the bone by the clot and significant venous bleeding was seen at the area of the sinus. This was controlled with Gelfoam soaked in thrombin held in place by cottonoid strips and gentle pressure. A high-speed drill was used to make suture tack-up holes on either side of the strip of bone over the sinus. Tack-up sutures were placed in the dura superior and inferior to the strip of bone, passed through the drill holes, and secured in place over strips of Gelfoam placed longitudinally along both sides of the bony bridge. After ensuring there was no more bleeding from the bony edges, the occipital and the posterior fossa bone flaps were replaced and the wound was closed.

There are several surgical techniques and nuances used to manage dural venous sinus injuries. Preferring one technique over another largely depends on intraoperative circumstances and assessment of the degree of the venous sinus injury. This may also vary based on the neurosurgeon's preference and expertise. Applying pressure with a Gelfoam pad and cottonoid patties is a commonly used technique to initially tamponade and stop the bleeding. Thrombin in the Gelfoam helps induce coagulation. Gelfoam may sometimes be left in place in the epidural space. Over-sewing with a muscle patch or packing with Surgicel are other techniques that may be used in some cases. Direct suturing of the sinus can be performed, as well as direct repair of the roof of the sinus with pericranium or fascia. If the bleeding is controlled by tamponade, this may not be necessary. For uncontrolled venous sinus bleeding, direct repair must be done with able assistants who are capable of providing simultaneous pressure to stave off bleeding, flooding of the field with irrigation, and suctioning of blood for visualization. Rarely, a completely transected dural venous sinus may need to be ligated to avoid massive blood loss. While this technique may be tolerated in some cases, it can be associated with significant morbidity and mortality secondary to severe venous congestion, elevated intracranial pressure, and possibly large venous infarction.

While many neurosurgeons would agree that exposing both sides of the transverse sinus is necessary in evacuating an EDH in a case like the one presented, the strategy of leaving an intact piece of bone over the area of the sinus has advantages. It may allow the surgeon to avoid directly manipulating an injured venous sinus, thus avoiding excessive bleeding, and it provides a bony rim on which to secure tack-up sutures to help tamponade the bleeding. The two craniotomies (occipital and suboccipital) created on each side of the venous sinus are usually enough to allow complete evacuation of the hematoma.

In addition to intraoperative venous sinus bleeding concerns, which can be difficult to control, a venous sinus laceration is associated with the risk of an air embolus. It is therefore important to inform the anesthesiologist of this concern and to use intraoperative Doppler ultrasound (to hear) or an echocardiogram probe (to see) the embolism in the heart if possible. Copious irrigation during the procedure and avoiding the sitting position may reduce the risk of an air embolus. Signs of air embolism include hypotension and hypoxia, and, if suspected, there are key maneuvers that should be done immediately, namely flooding the field with continuous, copious irrigation, and placing the patient immediately into the left lateral decubitus position in order to trap the air bubble in the right atrium so it can be evacuated through a central line. In case of cardiac arrest, chest compressions can result in fragmentation of large air bubbles in the right ventricular chamber, obstructing blood flow.

Oral Boards Review: Management Pearls

- Suspicion of a venous sinus injury may prompt the surgeon to approach the lesion with a bone flap on either side of the EDH so as to leave a strip of bone to tamponade bleeding and to which to secure tack-up sutures
- Make certain that the anesthesia team is aware of the possibility of air embolism, and monitors carefully for signs.
- If a sinus injury is present, blood loss may be significant, and the surgical team should be prepared to transfuse blood products as necessary.

Pivot Points

- If the patient presents in coma with anisocoria or if the EDH is greater than 30 cc in volume, plan for emergent surgical evacuation.
- If the EDH involves the posterior fossa, consider early evacuation.
- In general, the simplest and safest control of bleeding from a venous sinus is with hemostatic agents and pressure. If bleeding is controlled, tack the dura and close.

Aftercare

The most common and concerning complication after surgery is rebleeding. The risk of rebleeding is thought to be higher in EDH from venous sinus injury as compared to EDH of other etiology. Rebleeding can significantly increase the morbidity and mortality. Close monitoring in an intensive care unit setting after surgery is crucial and is recommended to allow for prompt detection of any neurological change. The patient in this case was kept intubated after the procedure and was transferred to the intensive care unit for continuous monitoring of vital signs and hourly neurological examinations. An overnight, routine postoperative CT scan of the brain was obtained and showed expected postcraniotomy findings, evacuated EDH, and no evidence of rebleeding. Clinically, the patient was following commands in all four extremities and was extubated on postoperative day 1. The Jackson Pratt drain was removed on the same day, and patient was discharged on day 5 after surgery.

Complications and Management

As previously discussed, massive intraoperative bleeding is a potential complication of the surgical management of dural venous sinus injury. Commonly used techniques for stopping sinus bleeding were discussed in detail in the "Surgical Procedure" section. In brief, techniques to stop sinus bleeding may include applying a Gelfoam pad over the bleeding site, reinforcing and packing with Surgicel, directly suturing the venous sinus with stitches if technically feasible, using a patch graft of pericranium or fascia for an avulsed part of the sinus wall, or complete ligation of the sinus as a final resort. Postoperative bleeding is another potential complication that may require reoperation.

Air embolism is a rare but well-known complication of the surgical management of venous sinus injury that is associated with significant morbidity and mortality. Early recognition and rapid intervention during surgery can be life-saving. Air embolism occurs as a result of direct communication between the atmosphere and the venous system. Suctioning of air into the dural venous sinuses can lead to transmission of an air embolus to the heart and then the pulmonary artery. It is therefore important to discuss this potential risk with the anesthesiologist prior to surgery and use intraoperative Doppler to detect any signs of air embolism. Copious irrigation of the opening in the sinus during repair may reduce the risk of air embolism. Avoiding the sitting position may also reduce the risk. The clinical signs of air embolism may include bradycardia and hypotension that are nonresponsive to treatment, oxygen desaturations and reduced end tidal carbon dioxide levels, and cardiac arrest, or it may be clinically silent but detected using a precordial Doppler ultrasound or bedside echocardiogram probe.

Once an air embolism is detected, the next immediate technical maneuver would be to close any potential conduit between the atmosphere and the venous sinuses. This may be achieved by asking the first assistant to copiously irrigate the wound or by applying hemostatic agents or a wet lap sponge over any open communication to the sinus. Positioning the patient in a Trendelenburg position (Durant's maneuver) may help relieve the "air-lock" effect on the right ventricle and thus prevent a cardiopulmonary shock. Putting the patient in the left lateral decubitus position is also indicated; however, if this maneuver is hindered by positioning (e.g., if the patient is prone and/or in the Mayfield three-pin headholder), the position can be approximated by rotating the table, taking care to keep the patient securely positioned on the operating table. Achieving hemostasis and wound closure should be performed quickly if the patient is clinically symptomatic. In case of hemodynamic instability, chest compressions should be started and routine application of advanced cardiac life support should be initiated. Cardiac bypass may even be required. Hyperbaric oxygen therapy plays an important role in the management of air embolism, especially in patients with evidence of neurological or any other end-organ damage.

Oral Boards Review: Complications Pearls

- Surveillance for possible rehemorrhage is important.
- Maintain a high suspicion for possibility of intraoperative air embolism.

Evidence and Outcomes

Clinical data regarding injuries to the venous sinuses are principally from case series and case reports. The outcome of patients with EDH depends on several factors. These may include the presenting GCS score, the overall traumatic burden and other injuries, age, and medical comorbidities, as well as intra- and postoperative complications. The preoperative neurological status of the patient is thought to be the best predictor of outcome, and an early surgical intervention is associated with overall better outcome.

Further Reading

Bullock MR, Chesnut R, Ghajar J, et al. Surgical management of acute epidural hematomas. *Neurosurgery*. 2006;58(3 Suppl):S7–15; discussion Si–iv. https://www.ncbi.nlm.nih.gov/pubmed/16710967

Fernandes-Cabral DT, Kooshkabadi A, Panesar SS, et al. Surgical management of vertex epidural hematoma: Technical case report and literature review. *World Neurosurg*. 2017;103:475–483. https://www.ncbi.nlm.nih.gov/pubmed/28427975

Lapadula G, Caporlingua F, Paolini S, Missori P, Domenicucci M. Epidural hematoma with detachment of the dural sinuses. *J Neurosci Rural Pract*. 2014;5(2):191–194. https://www.ncbi.nlm.nih.gov/pubmed/24966568

McCarthy CJ, Behravesh S, Naidu SG, Oklu R. Air embolism: Diagnosis, clinical management and outcomes. *Diagnostics (Basel)*. 2017;7(1). https://www.ncbi.nlm.nih.gov/pubmed/28106717

Yilmazlar S, Kocaeli H, Dogan S, et al. Traumatic epidural haematomas of nonarterial origin: analysis of 30 consecutive cases. *Acta Neurochir (Wien)*. 2005;147(12):1241–1248; discussion 1248. https://www.ncbi.nlm.nih.gov/pubmed/16133767

Traumatic Intracerebral Contusions

Ilyas Eli, Mitchell Couldwell, and Craig H. Rabb

7

Case Presentation

A 22-year-old man with past medical history significant for type I diabetes presented to the emergency department (ED) after falling from a 6-foot ladder. As he fell, he hit his head on an adjacent building and subsequently lost consciousness. He was transported to the ED as a trauma patient. On neurological examination, he had a Glasgow Coma Scale (GCS) score of 13 (spontaneous eye opening, confused on verbal response, and localized motor response to pain). His pupils were reactive, his face appeared symmetric, and he moved all of his extremities. Noncontrast CT scans demonstrated bilateral inferior frontal hemorrhagic contusions with associated cerebral edema (Figure 7.1).

Questions

1. Where should the patient be admitted?
2. What is the pathophysiology of intracerebral contusions?
3. What regions of the brain are susceptible to contusion formation?

Assessment and Planning

The patient was admitted to the neurocritical care unit (NCCU) for the management of his traumatic brain injury (TBI). He was closely monitored every hour with neurological examinations. He was also started on levetiracetam for seizure prophylaxis. His neurological findings improved and he had a GCS of 15 in the NCCU. A repeat CT scan performed 6 h after the initial scan demonstrated "blossoming" of his cerebral contusions, but another repeat CT scan 6 h later showed a stable appearance of the bifrontal contusions.

Oral Boards Review: Diagnostic Pearls

- A comprehensive assessment of clinical findings and imaging characteristics is important for determining whether surgical or nonsurgical management is appropriate:
  - GCS score at admission is an important indicator of patient status.
  - Patients with intracranial contusions should be monitored in the neurocritical care unit.

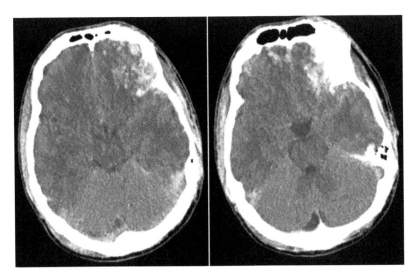

Figure 7.1 Axial CT scan of the brain without contrast enhancement demonstrates inferior bifrontal hemorrhagic contusions with associated cerebral edema.

- CT scan of the brain is the imaging modality of choice for visualizing and monitoring contusions.
- Contusions will develop edema over time and commonly can undergo hemorrhagic progression.
- Patients should be monitored for hyponatremia, which can worsen neurological examination findings and can result in exacerbation of cerebral edema.

TBI is a major cause of death, disability, and socioeconomic burden worldwide.[1,2] Traumatic intracerebral contusions are a subtype of TBI akin to a bruise on the surface of the brain. Cerebral contusions are present in 13–35% of patients who incur a TBI, classically as a result of coup or contrecoup injuries in motor vehicle accidents and falls.[3–5] Contusions frequently develop as a result of direct traumatic impact of the brain against the inner table of the skull or sliding against a bony ridge at the cranial base. The impact results in injury to capillaries, which results in small petechial hemorrhages. The lesion involves the gray and white matter and can be nonhemorrhagic, have microhemorrhages, or can be grossly hemorrhagic. Over time, contusions will develop mass effect from vasogenic or cytotoxic edema, presumably as a result of hyperosmolarity in the center of the contusion generating an osmotic gradient and attraction of water into the contusion.[6] Contusions are commonly located along the poles and inferior frontal, temporal, and occipital surfaces.[7] CT is the preferred imaging tool utilized for detection and assessment of intracranial hematomas. CT scans show an area of hyperdense hemorrhage or heterogenous density along with a peripheral rim of low density due to associated vasogenic edema. MRI can be obtained; it will show a T2 hypointense lesion with surrounding edema that is hyperintense on fluid-attenuated inversion recovery (FLAIR) and T2 sequences. On imaging, the contusions can have a range of appearances ranging from a solid hematoma to a patchy appearance.[2] It is common for cerebral contusions to increase in size and undergo hemorrhagic progression on repeated imaging as a result of edema and hematoma expansion, which occurs in 38–59% of cases. Because of this hemorrhagic progression, serial imaging is necessary to assess changes.[8,9]

Questions

1. Which brain lobes are susceptible to contusion formation?
2. What is a concern with temporal lobe contusions?

Decision Making

The severity of patient status is based on initial GCS score, which can range from mild (GCS = 13–15) to severe (GCS ≤8) injury. Our patient had an initial GCS score of 13, which is why placement of an intracranial pressure (ICP) monitoring device was not pursued. The Brain Trauma Foundation's guideline for management of TBI suggests placement of an ICP monitoring device in patients with GCS score of 3–8 after resuscitation with an abnormal CT findings or GCS score of 3–8 with a normal scan if two or more of the following criteria are met: age greater than 40 years, episode of hypotension (blood pressure <90 mm Hg), and/or abnormal motor response (motor posturing).[10]

Questions

1. What are the indications for surgical intervention?
2. What are the surgical options?

Surgical intervention is indicated in patients with clinical deterioration of neurological examination findings, refractory ICPs after exhaustive medical management, or imaging findings of mass effect. Furthermore, patients with GCS score of 6–8 with a frontal or temporal contusion that has a volume greater than 20 cm³ with a midline shift of 5 mm or more and/or cisternal compression or contusion greater than 50 cm³ should undergo surgical treatment. Surgery entails a craniotomy with evacuation of the contusion to relieve elevated ICP and brain shift. However, the location of the lesion in relation to critical structures should be kept in mind. In patients with diffuse unilateral or bilateral contusion, a decompressive hemicraniectomy or a bifrontal decompressive craniectomy can be performed.[11]

Because of our patient's good findings on clinical examination, with no significant signs of mass effect on imaging, we pursued nonsurgical management. The patient's medical management consisted of close observation, repeat imaging at 6-h intervals until a stable scan was achieved, levetiracetam for seizure prophylaxis, and systolic blood pressure maintenance of above 110 mm Hg. The patient's neurological examination findings continued to improve. He was transferred to the regular floor on hospital day 3. He was discharged on hospital day 6 to an inpatient rehabilitation facility.

On day 2 of his stay in the rehabilitation facility, the patient was noted to have an acute mental status decline with a GCS of 10. He underwent repeat imaging of his brain, which showed increased cerebral edema with midline shift (Figure 7.2). He

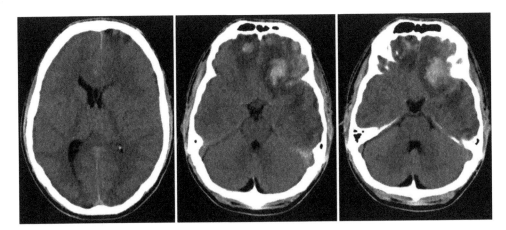

Figure 7.2 Axial CT scan of the brain without contrast enhancement demonstrates bilateral inferior frontal hemorrhagic contusions, left greater than right, with surrounding edema. The degree of edema has increased with left lateral ventricle effacement and midline shift measuring 7 mm.

also had a sodium level of 126 mEq/L. He was readmitted to the NCCU for further management. Salt supplementation was initiated with salt tablets and hypertonic saline. The patient's GCS score improved to 15 a day later, and he was discharged home with outpatient therapies after another 8 days of hospital stay. He was seen in clinic for follow-up 1 month after discharge from the hospital. The patient reported satisfactory cognitive function, including appropriate short-term memory and word-finding ability. His parents reported that he had been irritable after the injury, but that his demeanor was normalized now. On examination, he was awake, alert, and fluently conversant. He walked with an upright posture and a swift and steady gait. CT of the brain without contrast showed resolution of the bifrontal contusions (Figure 7.3).

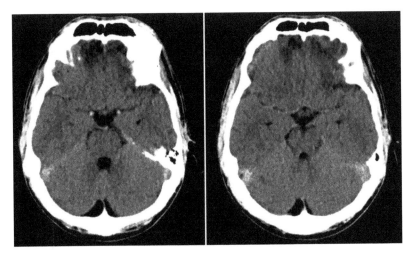

Figure 7.3 Axial CT scan of the brain without contrast enhancement demonstrates resolution of the contusion involving the inferior frontal lobes.

Oral Boards Review: Management Pearls

- An ICP monitoring device should be placed in patients with GCS score 8 or lower.
- Surgery entails a craniotomy with evacuation of hematoma, but if there is a diffuse focus of contusion, then a hemicraniectomy or a bifrontal craniectomy can be performed.

Pivot Points

- Contusions can commonly undergo hemorrhagic progression. Patients should be monitored closely, and any neurological changes should warrant repeat imaging.
- Temporal lobe contusions can herniate without changes in ICP.

Aftercare

Aftercare of patients with cerebral contusion will vary depending on whether surgical or nonsurgical management is used. Patients are monitored in the NCCU for several days until their neurological examination findings improve and stable imaging is obtained. In the NCCU, continuous blood pressure is monitored and serial neurological examinations are performed. The patient is also evaluated by the physical medicine and rehabilitation team for rehabilitation candidacy.

Patients who undergo decompressive craniectomy require further postoperative imaging and neurocritical care monitoring. An ICP monitor is essential to ensure ICP is lowered after surgery and to monitor for ICP elevations due to postoperative edema or new hematoma formation. Postoperatively, the patient's head is positioned facing toward the contralateral side, and a helmet is placed. Patients are monitored for early, late, and delayed complications related to decompressive craniectomy. Replacement of the bone flap is planned for a later date several months after the craniectomy.

Complications and Management

Hyponatremia

Hyponatremia occurs commonly in patients with intracranial injury and must be closely monitored. The incidence is quoted in the literature to range from 9.6% to 51%.[12,13] Hyponatremia results in exacerbation of cerebral edema, which can result in worsening of neurological outcome.[14] The two most common causes of hyponatremia in patients with head injury are cerebral salt wasting (CSW) and syndrome of inappropriate antidiuretic hormone secretion (SIADH); other potential causes are inadequate intake of salt and pituitary dysfunction. Patients with head injury should be monitored for hyponatremia with daily sodium checks and more frequent checks if hyponatremia is found. An attempt should be made to diagnose the cause of the hyponatremia, although this can be challenging. Treatment options mentioned in the literature include fluid restriction, dietary salt supplementation, and use of fludrocortisone. The initial attempt to treat hyponatremia should involve salt supplementation and hydration, but if that does not correct serum sodium, fluid restriction is a possible treatment option. Fluid restriction should be used judiciously because dehydrating TBI patients can result in adverse outcome. Dringer et al.[15] showed that patients with SIADH treated with fluid restriction are at a higher risk for delayed neurological deficits. In a retrospective study of 1,500 TBI patients, Rajagopal et al.[16] found that 13.2% of patients had hyponatremia and noted that early initiation of fludrocortisone is associated with a shorter hospital stay. Early use of salt supplementation and salt-retaining therapy should be used for treatment of hyponatremia in TBI patients, while fluid restriction should be used judiciously.

Hemorrhagic Progression of Contusion

Contusions can blossom over time, a condition called *hemorrhagic progression of contusion* (HPC). Half of patients with contusions demonstrate HPC, manifested by a change in neurological findings. Furthermore, in patients with no worsening of their neurological examination, 15% can have evidence of HPC.[17,18] HPC occurs within the first 12 h but can occur in a delayed fashion up to several days after initial presentation. Patients with temporal lobe contusions need to be monitored closely for HPC. The contusion in the medial portion of the temporal lobe is located close to the tentorium and can result in mass effect with contusion swelling in the direction of the tentorial notch and even uncal herniation without an increase in ICP. Surgical decompression may be required in temporal contusions that are noted to increase in size on repeat imaging.

Surgical Complications and Management

Decompressive craniectomy is effective for decreasing ICP, but it is not without risks. Postoperative complications include contusion expansion, seizures, subdural effusion, CSF leak, delayed hydrocephalus, syndrome of the trephined, and postoperative infection. After decompressive craniectomy, contusion expansion can result from changing ICP dynamics due to loss of tamponade from bone removal, which may result in an increase in the size of the contusion.[19] Close observation is required to monitor the contusion expansion. Seizures can occur; however, they can potentially be prevented with prophylactic antiepileptic medication. External cerebral herniation can be due to cerebral edema and can cause cortical vein compression via entrapment against the bone edge, which can result in venous infarction. During the decompressive craniectomy, a wide craniectomy allows for cerebral edema without cortical vein compression. Some patients can develop a CSF leak, but this is uncommon. Subdural effusion formation is a delayed complication caused by disruption of the dura and arachnoid. These generally resolve spontaneously over time without surgical intervention but should be monitored. Postoperative infection can be treated with antibiotics. Delayed hydrocephalus, which presents with ventriculomegaly, develops as a result of alteration in CSF flow. Hydrocephalus is treated with ventriculoperitoneal shunt placement. Syndrome of the trephined is a long-term phenomenon that occurs after the scalp sinks into the bone defect and exerts atmospheric pressure on the underlying brain, resulting in symptoms of headaches and seizures. Treatment for syndrome of the trephine is to replace the bone via cranioplasty.[19]

Oral Boards Review: Complications Pearls

- What are the common complications associated with a decompressive hemicraniectomy?
- How are postoperative subdural effusions managed?

Evidence and Outcomes

Recovery after a brain contusion varies widely, and outcomes depend patient age, initial GCS score, and the size and location of the contusion. Studies suggest that cerebral contusions are associated with overall worse clinical course and higher mortality.[18,20] Alahmadi et al.[2] performed a retrospective study to investigate the factors that predict radiographic and clinical progression of contusions in patients who were managed nonoperatively. Their results demonstrated that 45% of cerebral contusions managed conservatively progressed radiographically over time, with 19% eventually requiring surgical intervention. Furthermore, their data show that older patients with worse GCS score and patients with large contusions and subdural hematoma tend to have contusion expansion. The presence of a brain contusion predicted whether patients with TBI complained of memory and emotional changes since the frontal lobe is involved in working and long-term memory processing.[21] Huang et al.[22] performed a retrospective study evaluating the surgical treatment of hemorrhagic cerebral contusion via craniotomy with evacuation of hematoma in 16 patients or decompressive craniectomy in 38 patients. The craniectomy group had a significantly lower Glasgow Outcome Scale-Extended score, lower reoperation rate, lower mortality rate (13.2% vs. 25%), and lower reoperation rate (7.9% vs. 37.5%). A randomized controlled trial evaluating the use of oral glibenclamide (also known as glyburide), an antidiabetic drug, was associated with decreased expansion of cerebral contusion in patients with TBI, although glibenclamide did not improve functional outcomes.[23] Another randomized trial demonstrated no change in contusion size when patients were treated with atorvastatin, but showed that patients had improvement in functional outcomes (measured on the Glasgow Outcome Scale, modified Rankin scale, and Disability Rating Scale) at 3 months after injury.[24]

References

1. Iaccarino C, Schiavi P, Picetti E, et al. Patients with brain contusions: Predictors of outcome and relationship between radiological and clinical evolution. *J Neurosurg.* 2014;120(4):908–918.
2. Alahmadi H, Vachhrajani S, Cusimano MD. The natural history of brain contusion: An analysis of radiological and clinical progression. *J Neurosurg.* 2010;112(5):1139–1145.
3. Bullock R, Golek J, Blake G. Traumatic intracerebral hematoma: Which patients should undergo surgical evacuation? CT scan features and ICP monitoring as a basis for decision making. *Surg Neurol.* 1989;32(3):181–187.

4. Carnevale JA, Segar DJ, Powers AY, et al. Blossoming contusions: Identifying factors contributing to the expansion of traumatic intracerebral hemorrhage. *J Neurosurg.* 2018:1–12.

5. Lobato RD, Cordobes F, Rivas JJ, et al. Outcome from severe head injury related to the type of intracranial lesion. A computerized tomography study. *J Neurosurg.* 1983;59(5):762–774.

6. Kawamata T, Mori T, Sato S, Katayama Y. Tissue hyperosmolality and brain edema in cerebral contusion. *Neurosurg Focus.* 2007;22(5):E5.

7. Hijaz TA, Cento EA, Walker MT. Imaging of head trauma. *Radiol Clin North Am.* 2011;49(1):81–103.

8. Cepeda S, Gomez PA, Castano-Leon AM, Martinez-Perez R, Munarriz PM, Lagares A. Traumatic intracerebral hemorrhage: Risk factors associated with progression. *J Neurotrauma.* 2015;32(16):1246–1253.

9. Servadei F, Nanni A, Nasi MT, et al. Evolving brain lesions in the first 12 hours after head injury: Analysis of 37 comatose patients. *Neurosurgery.* 1995;37(5):899–906; discussion 906–897.

10. Carney N, Totten AM, O'Reilly C, et al. Guidelines for the management of severe traumatic brain injury, fourth edition. *Neurosurgery.* 2017;80(1):6–15.

11. Bullock MR, Chesnut R, Ghajar J, et al. Surgical management of traumatic parenchymal lesions. *Neurosurgery.* 2006;58(3 Suppl):S25–46; discussion Si-iv.

12. Sherlock M, O'Sullivan E, Agha A, et al. Incidence and pathophysiology of severe hyponatraemia in neurosurgical patients. *Postgrad Med J.* 2009;85(1002):171–175.

13. Yumoto T, Sato K, Ugawa T, Ichiba S, Ujike Y. Prevalence, risk factors, and short-term consequences of traumatic brain injury-associated hyponatremia. *Acta Med Okayama.* 2015;69(4):213–218.

14. Gray JR, Morbitzer KA, Liu-DeRyke X, Parker D, Zimmerman LH, Rhoney DH. Hyponatremia in patients with spontaneous intracerebral hemorrhage. *J Clin Med.* 2014;3(4):1322–1332.

15. Diringer MN, Zazulia AR. Hyponatremia in neurologic patients: Consequences and approaches to treatment. *Neurologist.* 2006;12(3):117–126.

16. Rajagopal R, Swaminathan G, Nair S, Joseph M. Hyponatremia in traumatic brain injury: A practical management protocol. *World Neurosurg.* 2017;108:529–533.

17. Sifri ZC, Homnick AT, Vaynman A, et al. A prospective evaluation of the value of repeat cranial computed tomography in patients with minimal head injury and an intracranial bleed. *J Trauma.* 2006;61(4):862–867.

18. Oertel M, Kelly DF, McArthur D, et al. Progressive hemorrhage after head trauma: Predictors and consequences of the evolving injury. *J Neurosurg.* 2002;96(1):109–116.

19. Kurland DB, Khaladj-Ghom A, Stokum JA, et al. Complications associated with decompressive craniectomy: A systematic review. *Neurocrit Care.* 2015;23(2):292–304.

20. Kurland D, Hong C, Aarabi B, Gerzanich V, Simard JM. Hemorrhagic progression of a contusion after traumatic brain injury: a review. *J Neurotrauma.* 2012;29(1):19–31.

21. Su BY, Guo NW, Chen NC, et al. Brain contusion as the main risk factor of memory or emotional complaints in chronic complicated mild traumatic brain injury. *Brain Inj.* 2017;31(5):601–606.

22. Huang AP, Tu YK, Tsai YH, et al. Decompressive craniectomy as the primary surgical intervention for hemorrhagic contusion. *J Neurotrauma.* 2008;25(11):1347–1354.

23. Khalili H, Derakhshan N, Niakan A, et al. Effects of oral glibenclamide on brain contusion volume and functional outcome of patients with moderate and severe traumatic brain

injuries: A randomized double-blind placebo-controlled clinical trial. *World Neurosurg.* 2017;101:130–136.

24. Farzanegan GR, Derakhshan N, Khalili H, Ghaffarpasand F, Paydar S. Effects of atorvastatin on brain contusion volume and functional outcome of patients with moderate and severe traumatic brain injury: A randomized double-blind placebo-controlled clinical trial. *J Clin Neurosci.* 2017;44:143–147.

Diffuse Axonal Injury

Hussein A. Zeineddine, Cole T. Lewis, and Ryan S. Kitagawa

8

Case Presentation

A 30-year-old man was involved in an automobile versus pedestrian accident and was unresponsive on scene. He was intubated at the scene. On arrival to the hospital, he was noted to have sluggishly reactive pupils, no movement to noxious stimuli, and a pulseless left lower extremity.

Questions

1. What is the likely diagnosis?
2. What is the most appropriate workup?
3. What is the most appropriate imaging modality at this time?

Assessment and Planning

The patient had a high-energy injury, so adequate resuscitation is paramount and is a priority over the patient's neurological condition. Advanced Trauma Life Support (ATLS) criteria require securing the airway and maintaining hemodynamic stability. The neurological assessment is then performed, followed by a secondary survey of other injuries. Based on this assessment, laboratory tests as well as imaging are obtained. This particular patient had a noncontrast head CT, cervical spine CT, CT angiography of the neck, and a CT chest/abdomen/pelvis/lower extremity. The head CT (Figure 8.1) revealed multiple hemorrhagic shearing injuries throughout the cerebral hemispheres. The left lower extremity CT demonstrated a femoral artery dissection.

Based on his clinical exam, the patient sustained a severe traumatic brain injury (TBI), which may include focal lesions such as contusions and extra-axial hematomas as well as diffuse lesions such as diffuse axonal injury (DAI). Adams was the first to use the term DAI in 1982,[1] but Strich first reported the white matter histopathological appearance after severe TBI in 1956.[2] Although no treatment is currently available, the severity of DAI has been shown to correlate with TBI outcomes in clinical and experimental observations.[3-5] DAI should be suspected when a high-energy injury occurs with a poor neurological exam.

The clinical presentation of DAI is typically out of proportion to the CT findings, and the degree of neurological compromise is related to the severity of the axonal insult. Mild DAI reflects a concussive disorder with headache as the most common symptom. However, severe DAI may include loss of consciousness, coma, and prolonged vegetative

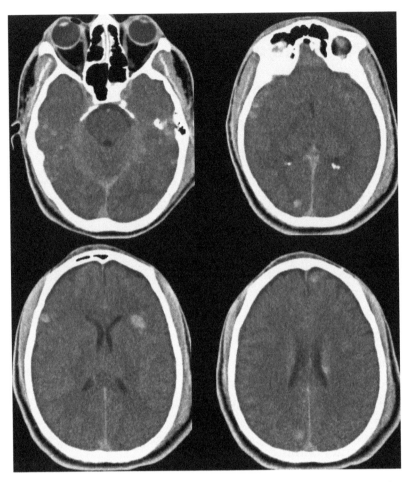

Figure 8.1 Computed tomography (CT) showing the typical DAI lesions. These are hemorrhagic lesions that appear hyperdense on CT scans. The severity of DAI is underestimated on CT scans as there can by small punctate lesions as well as non-hemorrhagic lesions. Affected areas still include the grey-white matter interface as well as the corpus callosum.

state or cognitive impairment. In the acute phase, decreased level of consciousness or coma is usually the result of DAI in the brainstem and/or diencephalon with resultant pathological changes including axonal swelling and Wallerian degeneration.[6] Regardless of the suspicion of DAI, the patient should be managed similar to any severe TBI, including resuscitation and neurological monitoring. In this particular patient, an intra-cranial pressure (ICP) monitor was placed, and he was taken to the operating room for treatment of the femoral artery injury.

Oral Boards Review: Diagnostic Pearls

- Management of a trauma should proceed with the ATLS algorithm.
- CT is the initial imaging modality to be obtained in the setting of trauma.
- TBI is a heterogenous disease including a variety of injuries, such as contusions, hematomas, and DAI.

DAI should be suspected based on the mechanism of presentation and if CT findings cannot fully explain the patient's exam, but this condition should be initially treated similar to all severe TBI.

Questions

1. What is the treatment for DAI?
2. What imaging modalities are available for diagnosis of DAI?

Decision Making

Once DAI is suspected, classifying and localizing DAI lesions may help in determining the patient's prognosis. However, the standard treatment of this condition will involve a number of modalities including ICP monitoring, cerebral blood flow (CBF) and brain oxygenation monitoring, EEG, neuroimaging, and fluid biomarkers. Neuroimaging is the best tool for diagnosis of DAI.

Computed Tomography

In the setting of trauma, a noncontrast head CT is the first-line imaging modality utilized. While essential for life-threatening and surgically amenable lesions, CT lacks adequate sensitivity for DAI. In one study of mild TBI, up to 30% of patients with normal brain imaging have MRI lesions of any nature within 2 weeks of trauma, which was associated with worse outcome.[7] When present on CT, lesions include small punctate hemorrhages/hyperdensities along white matter tracts with typical locations including the corpus callosum and the brainstem. When lesions are present on CT, this may reflect a more severe DAI.

Magnetic Resonance Imaging

MRI is the modality of choice for diagnosing DAI as this study may confirm the presence of micro hemorrhages in the white matter of the cerebral hemispheres, corpus callosum, and brainstem. Of the different sequences available, susceptibility weighted imaging (SWI) and T2★-weighted gradient echo (T2★GRE) are preferred for detecting micro hemorrhages, with SWI being more sensitive in deep-seated lesions such as the brainstem. Due to the presence of paramagnetic hemoglobin degradation products, the lesions appear as hypointense foci, but they appear larger than their true size due to the "blooming" effect from magnetic field distortion. The lesions decrease over time, and those identified on SWI appear to correlate with outcome more than on T2★GRE.

DAI can also present with nonhemorrhagic lesions, such as local edema associated with axonal injury. Fluid-attenuated inversion recovery (FLAIR) sequence and diffusion-weighted imaging (DWI) can detect such lesions. Although the FLAIR sequence is useful for identifying lesions in periventricular white matter, the corpus callosum, and the brainstem, DWI is more sensitive for detecting nonhemorrhagic injuries. Lesions on DWI may correlate with initial Glasgow Coma Scale (GCS) score and coma duration. However, both sequences are time-dependent as the lesions start to disappear by 3 months after injury.

Other neuroimaging techniques being studied include diffuse tensor imaging (DTI), magnetic resonance spectroscopy (MRS), single-photon emission computed tomography (SPECT), and positron emission tomography (PET). MRS provides information regarding neurochemical alterations.[8] Correlation with outcomes are unclear at this time; however, this imaging modality may have a promising future for use in prognostication. Vagnozzi et al. reported the use of MRS to monitor levels of N-acetylaspartate (NAA) after mild TBI and its utility in assessing brain vulnerability.[9] SPECT and PET sequences may provide value in evaluating the effects of DAI on physiological processes.

Currently, DTI has been shown to be the most effective in detecting DAI. DTI allows three-dimensional reconstruction of white matter tracts and quantitative assessment of injury. However, variation in data acquisition and post-processing as well as cost still limit the clinical applicability of many of these methods. Improvements in technology, standardization of sequencing, and cost reduction will likely make these advanced imaging modalities more commonplace in treatment of TBI patients.

Figure 8.2 shows that patient's MRI with the different sequences of T1, T2, T2 FLAIR, and SWI.

Questions

1. What are typical locations for DAI?
2. What are the classification systems available for DAI, and do those correlate with outcome?
3. What is the utility of fluid biomarkers in DAI?

Fluid Biomarkers

There are extensive studies in the literature investigating compounds, both in blood and CSF, in DAI. These compounds include neurofilaments, tau, spectrin breakdown proteins, amyloid precursor protein, and many others. Raheja et al. demonstrated that glial fibrillary acidic protein may predict both poor outcomes and long-term mortality.[10] However, none of these biomarkers is currently used in clinical practice due to the limited sensitivity and specificity they offer. Other barriers include variable half-lives and limited test availability.

Classifications and Outcomes

In 1989, Adams et al.[1] defined and graded the structural features of DAI using a series of 122 cases. DAI was observed in 28% of their cases, and these authors classified DAI microscopically into three grades.

Grade 1: Histological evidence of axonal injury is present in the white matter of the cerebral hemispheres, corpus callosum, brainstem, and, less commonly, the cerebellum.

Grade 2: A focal lesion in the corpus callosum also exists.

Grade 3: There is in addition a focal lesion in the dorsolateral quadrant or quadrants of the rostral brainstem.

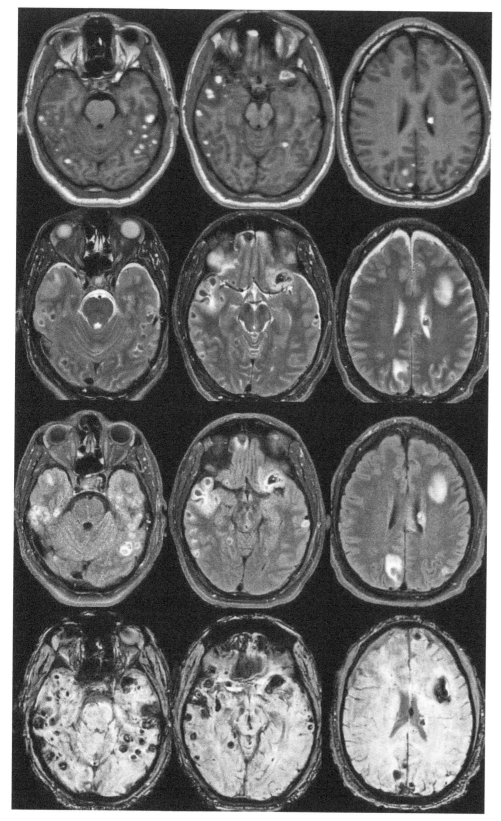

Figure 8.2 MRI images for above patient. T1-weighted (first row), T2-weighted (second row), FLAIR (third row) and SWI (last row) images. MR images reveals the true extent of the DAI which is under-represented on CT scans (Figure 1). MRI sequences, specifically SWI, is exquisitely sensitive in identifying DAI lesions. However, some lesions are non-hemorrhagic in nature and are better identified on FLAIR imaging. Lesions on SWI take longer to disappear compared to FLAIR imaging.

As histological studies are rarely available, DAI is usually diagnosed on MRI, and the modern grading system also has three grades.[11]

Grade 1: Traumatic lesions exist at the gray–white matter junction or lobar white matter or cerebellum only. Typical locations include parasagittal regions of frontal lobes, and the periventricular temporal lobes.

Grade 2: A corpus callosum lesion is present +/− grade 1.

Grade 3: Lesion are present in typical brainstem locations (dorsolateral quadrant of the upper brainstem, superior cerebellar peduncles) +/− grade 1 and 2.

Gennarelli et al. conducted controlled experiments in 45 monkeys by accelerating the head without impact in one of three directions.[3] These authors found that the duration of coma and degree of neurological impairment was proportional to the amount of DAI.

In two recent studies, the Adams DAI neuropathological grading did not linearly correlate with severity of outcome.[1,12] In one study, a lesion in the brainstem was associated with a worse outcome,[11] but DAI in other locations, such as corpus callosum, was not a negative prognostic factor. Another study also showed that brainstem lesions or substantia nigra lesions had an independent prognostic value, but grade 1 and 2 DAI lesions did not follow a linear increase in clinical severity.[13]

Other studies have shown that the greater the number of lesions observed early after trauma, the greater the impairment. Chastain et al. showed that the volume and number of lesions seen on MRI correlates with disability at discharge. For example, T2WI and FLAIR imaging were able to discriminate good and poor outcomes by median total lesion volume, median volume per lesion, and median number of lesions.[14] These findings were reproduced in other studies by Moen et al and Schaefer et al.[15, 16]

In a prospective study, of 19 patients, the number of MRI-based DAI lesions correlated with maximum ICP. Furthermore, patients with good outcome had fewer lesions and lower average maximum ICP.[17] Another study of 124 cases demonstrated that a DAI count of more than 6 is associated with poor outcome.[18] A more recent study examined MRI-defined DAI after TBI impact on functional outcomes, quality of life, and 3-year mortality. In a cohort of patients collected over 6 years, 56% had DAI, but no association was seen between DAI and long-term TBI outcomes.[19]

Surgical Procedure

There are limited therapeutic options for DAI. Currently, managing DAI is identical to the management of severe TBI and based on the Brain Trauma Foundation (BTF) Guidelines involves ICP management and maintenance of cerebral perfusion pressure. However, the presence of DAI alone does not necessarily correlate with increased ICP as the literature is variable, with some studies showing that maximum ICP correlates with the number of white matter lesions and others demonstrating that severe DAI patients did not have elevated ICP. Beyond the BTF guidelines for decreasing secondary insults, no acute management for the histopathological lesion in DAI is available.

There have been many well-planned clinical trials that have failed to show a benefit in the treatment of severe TBI. Multiple trials have used progesterone without improvement in clinical outcomes.[20,21] Hypothermia has been shown to reduce ICP when used in conjunction with standard care, but this did not result in improvement in long-term outcomes.[22] Continued research is needed to alleviate the large societal burden of TBI. At this time, repeated clinical examination and neuropsychological tests can provide valuable information on the extent of injury and prognosis, and early rehabilitation is essential.

Oral Boards Review: Management Pearls

- MRI is the imaging modality of choice for diagnosing DAI.
- Common locations for DAI include white matter of cerebral hemispheres, corpus callosum, and brainstem.
- A grading system was proposed by Adam et al., but recent evidence suggest that it does not fully predict outcome.
- Lesions in the brainstem have a negative prognostic value.
- DAI is the result of axonal stretching causing an insult to neuronal trafficking, which initiates a cascade of secondary events that include neuroinflammation, cytokine activation, and oxidative stress.
- Beyond ICP monitoring and optimizing cerebral perfusion pressure parameters, no acute management for the primary injury is available at this time.

Pivot Points

- If neurological injury is out of proportion to CT imaging findings, suspect underlying DAI.
- While there are no treatments specific to the DAI injury, treatment should be supportive care of the head-injured patient with attention directed at managing intracranial pressure.
- While there is no surgical treatment for DAI injuries, the patient may have other lesions such as subdural hematoma or epidural hematoma that require surgical treatment.

Questions

1. What are the mechanisms behind DAI?
2. How common is DAI compared to other forms of TBI?
3. What are the pathological bases for DAI?
4. How are various forms of DAI related to outcome?

Epidemiology/Etiology/Pathophysiology

A recent prospective study using MRI for diagnosing DAI demonstrated that DAI occurs in 72% of TBI cases (56% in moderate vs. 90% in severe TBI), with a pattern of "pure DAI" occurring in 22% of patients.[11] Other studies have cited a percentage of pure

DAI as low as 6%.[23] These studies have also shown that the more severe head injuries are associated with a higher frequency of DAI and of other concomitant lesions, and DAI is found in almost every fatal or very severe case of TBI. Although animal models have been developed to mimic open-head injuries as well as closed-head injuries, it remains difficult to fully replicate the forces in human DAI.[24,25]

TBI can manifest from focal injuries, such as an object striking the head resulting in skull fractures and localized hematomas, or from diffuse injuries such as DAI. DAI is the result of stretching and deformation of white matter tissue secondary to rapid rotational (angular) and/or linear (translational) acceleration-deceleration forces as would be seen with high-energy and high-velocity impacts, typically in road traffic accidents. This generates intracranial pressure gradients between the brain and skull that impart shear, tensile, and compressive strains on the brain. In such cases, the gray–white matter junction is most affected because the damage will be more evident in planes between tissues of different densities, as well as in the rostral brainstem given that it is the rotational center of mass. These forces need not cause a skull fracture or other intracranial injuries, but many times TBI may be the results of multiple forces resulting in a heterogeneous injury pattern.

While the initial event triggering DAI is defined, our understanding of the underlying pathophysiology remains incomplete. The initial impact imparts various forms of strains within the brain resulting in deformation of brain tissue. Using rat axons, it has been shown that not all axons sustain the same degree of injury, and certain axons are more vulnerable to brain injury, particularly in the unmyelinated white matter. Both the rate and magnitude of strain define the severity of axonal injury.

The rapid application of a strain prevents the brain from withstanding and adjusting to stretches and ultimately leads to deformation and disconnection between axons. However, primary axotomy is not the main mechanism behind DAI because delayed secondary axotomy is more frequently present. The details of the cellular and molecular pathways are beyond the scope of this chapter, but cytoskeletal alterations, particularly microtubules, seem to be one of the earliest changes detected. This results in failed axonal transport and accumulation of β-amyloid precursor protein (β-APP) with axonal swelling. Beyond that, secondary processes propagate the injury, including altered calcium homeostasis, activation of caspases and calpains, and, ultimately, necrosis and apoptosis. Studies have also shown that neuroinflammation, cytokine activation, oxidative stress, and reactive oxygen species contribute to axonal damage and neuronal death in DAI.

Multiple immunohistochemistry stains are useful in evaluation of DAI and include hematoxylin-eosin (H&E) staining, impregnation with silver, and β-APP, as well as others. However, β-APP is considered the gold standard as it has the ability to show axon damage very early after the brain injury. This is useful in cases of short survival time when damage is undetectable by H&E staining or impregnation with silver.[24–27]

Aftercare/Outcomes

In DAI survivors, the long-term effects include cognitive dysfunction and decreased quality of life from behavioral problems, as well as impairment in memory and executive

---

Oral Boards Review: Outcomes Pearls

- The lesion of DAI occurs frequently in the head-injured patient though it may coexist with other pathological conditions.
- Recovery from DAI is variable, though, in general, the more severe the initial injury, the less likely a favorable recovery.

---

functioning. Death rates among patients with DAI are generally between 20% and 30% at follow-up.[11,28] Of those remaining, there is a wide variety of reported outcomes. The most optimistic studies have an 88% recovery consistent with independent life and 12% of patients with dependence. However, most studies report worse outcomes with, frequency of disability and dependence ranging 40% to 88% and from 20% to 42%, respectively.

Factors that correlated with mortality at admission include pupillary changes, hypotension, hypoxia, and hyperglycemia. During hospitalization, GCS score after withdrawal of sedation and presence of intracerebral hemorrhage were associated with both mortality and dependence. Additionally, infection, continuous sedation time, and length of ICU stay were correlated with dependence.[28] For our particular patient, he required a tracheostomy and feeding tube immediately after the injury, but, following 3 months of rehabilitation, he was ambulatory without assistance and able to care for his basic activities of daily living. He is not functionally independent to date.

References

1. Adams JH, Doyle D, Ford I, Gennarelli TA, Graham DI, McLellan DR. Diffuse axonal injury in head injury: Definition, diagnosis and grading. *Histopathology*. Jul 1989;15(1):49–59.

2. Strich SJ. Diffuse degeneration of the cerebral white matter in severe dementia following head injury. *J Neurol Neurosurg Psychiatry*. Aug 1956;19(3):163–185.

3. Gennarelli TA, Thibault LE, Adams JH, Graham DI, Thompson CJ, Marcincin RP. Diffuse axonal injury and traumatic coma in the primate. *Ann Neurol*. Dec 1982;12(6):564–574.

4. Smith DH, Nonaka M, Miller R, et al. Immediate coma following inertial brain injury dependent on axonal damage in the brainstem. *J Neurosurg*. Aug 2000;93(2):315–322.

5. Magnoni S, Esparza TJ, Conte V, et al. Tau elevations in the brain extracellular space correlate with reduced amyloid-beta levels and predict adverse clinical outcomes after severe traumatic brain injury. *Brain*. Apr 2012;135(Pt 4):1268–1280.

6. McKee AC, Daneshvar DH. The neuropathology of traumatic brain injury. *Handb Clin Neurol*. 2015;127:45–66.

7. Yuh EL, Mukherjee P, Lingsma HF, et al. Magnetic resonance imaging improves 3-month outcome prediction in mild traumatic brain injury. *Ann Neurol*. Feb 2013;73(2):224–235.

8. Tsitsopoulos PP, Abu Hamdeh S, Marklund N. Current opportunities for clinical monitoring of axonal pathology in traumatic brain injury. *Front Neurol*. 2017;8:599.

9. Vagnozzi R, Signoretti S, Cristofori L, et al. Assessment of metabolic brain damage and recovery following mild traumatic brain injury: A multicentre, proton magnetic resonance spectroscopic study in concussed patients. *Brain*. Nov 2010;133(11):3232–3242.

10. Raheja A, Sinha S, Samson N, et al. Serum biomarkers as predictors of long-term outcome in severe traumatic brain injury: Analysis from a randomized placebo-controlled Phase II clinical trial. *J Neurosurg*. Sep 2016;125(3):631–641.

11. Skandsen T, Kvistad KA, Solheim O, Strand IH, Folvik M, Vik A. Prevalence and impact of diffuse axonal injury in patients with moderate and severe head injury: A cohort study of early magnetic resonance imaging findings and 1-year outcome. *J Neurosurg*. Sep 2010;113(3):556–563.

12. Adams JH, Graham DI, Murray LS, Scott G. Diffuse axonal injury due to nonmissile head injury in humans: An analysis of 45 cases. *Ann Neurol*. Dec 1982;12(6):557–563.

13. Abu Hamdeh S, Marklund N, Lannsjo M, et al. Extended anatomical grading in diffuse axonal injury using MRI: Hemorrhagic lesions in the substantia nigra and mesencephalic tegmentum indicate poor long-term outcome. *J Neurotrauma*. Jan 15 2017;34(2):341–352.

14. Chastain CA, Oyoyo UE, Zipperman M, et al. Predicting outcomes of traumatic brain injury by imaging modality and injury distribution. *J Neurotrauma*. Aug 2009;26(8):1183–1196.

15. Moen KG, Skandsen T, Folvik M, et al. A longitudinal MRI study of traumatic axonal injury in patients with moderate and severe traumatic brain injury. *J Neurol Neurosurg Psychiatry*. Dec 2012;83(12):1193–1200.

16. Schaefer PW, Huisman TA, Sorensen AG, Gonzalez RG, Schwamm LH. Diffusion-weighted MR imaging in closed head injury: High correlation with initial Glasgow Coma Scale score and score on modified Rankin scale at discharge. *Radiology*. Oct 2004;233(1):58–66.

17. Yanagawa Y, Sakamoto T, Takasu A, Okada Y. Relationship between maximum intracranial pressure and traumatic lesions detected by T2*-weighted imaging in diffuse axonal injury. *J Trauma*. Jan 2009;66(1):162–165.

18. Chelly H, Chaari A, Daoud E, et al. Diffuse axonal injury in patients with head injuries: An epidemiologic and prognosis study of 124 cases. *J Trauma*. Oct 2011;71(4):838–846.

19. Humble SS, Wilson LD, Wang L, et al. Prognosis of diffuse axonal injury with traumatic brain injury. *J Trauma Acute Care Surg*. Feb 17 2018;85(1):155–159.

20. Skolnick BE, Maas AI, Narayan RK, et al. A clinical trial of progesterone for severe traumatic brain injury. *N Engl J Med*. Dec 25 2014;371(26):2467–2476.

21. Wright DW, Yeatts SD, Silbergleit R, et al. Very early administration of progesterone for acute traumatic brain injury. *N Engl J Med*. Dec 25 2014;371(26):2457–2466.

22. Andrews PJ, Sinclair HL, Rodriguez A, et al. Hypothermia for intracranial hypertension after traumatic brain injury. *N Engl J Med*. Dec 17 2015;373(25):2403–2412.

23. Scheid R, Walther K, Guthke T, Preul C, von Cramon DY. Cognitive sequelae of diffuse axonal injury. *Arch Neurol*. Mar 2006;63(3):418–424.

24. Sharp DJ, Scott G, Leech R. Network dysfunction after traumatic brain injury. *Nat Rev Neurol*. Mar 2014;10(3):156–166.

25. Blennow K, Brody DL, Kochanek PM, et al. Traumatic brain injuries. *Nat Rev Dis Primers*. Nov 17 2016;2:16084.

26. Frati A, Cerretani D, Fiaschi AI, et al. Diffuse axonal injury and oxidative stress: A comprehensive review. *Int J Mol Sci*. Dec 2 2017;18(12).

27. Siedler DG, Chuah MI, Kirkcaldie MT, Vickers JC, King AE. Diffuse axonal injury in brain trauma: Insights from alterations in neurofilaments. *Front Cell Neurosci*. 2014;8:429.

28. Vieira RC, Paiva WS, de Oliveira DV, Teixeira MJ, de Andrade AF, de Sousa RM. Diffuse axonal injury: Epidemiology, outcome and associated risk factors. *Front Neurol*. 2016;7:178.

Concussion

Amy A. Mathews and Kathleen R. Bell

Our patient is a 41-year-old male dentist who, while playing in a recreational soccer game, attempted a header, made contact with an opponent, and subsequently fell to the ground. He lay motionless for approximately 1 min before attempting to sit himself upright with some clumsiness. The sideline physicians evaluated him on the field, cleared his cervical spine, and assisted him off the field to complete further evaluation. He reported minimal symptoms and was directed to the nearest emergency department.

Questions

1. What is the likely diagnosis?
2. How would you decide to remove the player from further play?
3. What evaluations would you perform on the sideline? When would you perform these evaluations?
4. Would you obtain any imaging?

Assessment and Planning

On-field assessment: The on-field assessment of an athlete with a suspected sports-related concussion (SRC) can be challenging. Interruption of competition, the athlete's wish to return to play, and chaotic testing conditions require a focused and skilled evaluator. The goal of the on-field assessment is to quickly determine if the athlete should be removed from play for a more thorough sideline evaluation. An athlete may be removed from play when there is an observed trauma with significant blow to the head or other hard body contact with subsequent deviation in behavior. Behavioral deviations that would warrant removal from play include lying motionless on the playing surface or exhibiting gait changes or labored movements, disorientation, a vacant stare, or facial injury due to the trauma. *Maddock's questions* (see Box 9.1) are used to assess orientation on-field because routine orientation questions have been shown to inadequately detect SRC. A Glasgow Coma Scale (GCS) score should be obtained. On-field assessments should also include a screen for any conditions that may prompt escalation of medical care, such as signs of cervical spine injury, focal neurological deficits, deteriorating consciousness, or seizure. It should be noted that loss of consciousness is not a definitive component of SRC, and many athletes may have minimal or mild symptoms upon immediate evaluation. A low threshold should be maintained to remove an athlete with suspected SRC from play—"when in doubt, sit them out."

Box 9.1 Maddock's Questions for Sports-Related Concussion

I am going to ask you a few questions, please listen carefully and give your best
    effort.
What venue are we at today?
Which half is it now?
Who scored last in this match?
What team did you play last week/game?
Did your team win the last game?

Sideline assessment: Once removed, the sideline assessment of the athlete with suspected
SRC should be systematic. Serial evaluations may be necessary because symptoms and
signs of SRC quickly change in the acute phase. There is no definitive examination, test,
biomarker, or imaging study with sufficient specificity to diagnose or exclude a concussion; instead, athletes should be evaluated in a comprehensive and methodical manner.
The sideline assessment should include a survey of symptoms and evaluations of mental
status, cognition, balance, and the nervous system.

The Standardized Assessment of Concussion (SAC) and the Sport Concussion
Assessment Tool – 5th edition (SCAT-5) are two resources used for sideline evaluation
of concussion. The SAC includes scored measures of orientation, memory, and concentration. Unscored portions of the SAC include a graded symptom checklist, documen-
tation of posttraumatic and/or retrograde amnesia, and a brief neurological exam. SAC
scores have been demonstrated to have good sensitivity and specificity when compared
with preinjury baseline scores. Concussed athletes have lower scores than nonconcussed
athletes, but there is no total score on the SAC that is diagnostic of concussion. Another
sideline evaluation tool, the SCAT-5 assessment, was revised in 2017 and is endorsed
by a consensus statement on concussion in sport. It is freely accessible and widely used
in the assessment of SRC. The SCAT5 is used for ages 13 and older and the pediatric
version (child SCAT5) for children 12 and under. The SCAT-5 sideline evaluation takes
approximately 10 min to administer and includes a symptom checklist, cognitive screen,
neurological screen, and Modified Balance Error Scoring System (mBESS) balance test.
The cognitive screen includes orientation, immediate and delayed memory, and concentration evaluations. Neurological screen includes assessments of speech, vision, cranial
nerves, coordination, strength, and gait. The mBESS tests balance through three different
stances over 20 sec with eyes closed. Cutoff scores diagnostic of concussion have not
been elucidated for either the SAC or SCAT-5, and these should be used as a tool in the
overall evaluation of the athlete with SRC.

Escalation of care: Evaluation of suspected SRC should be escalated to the ER setting
for any "red flag" symptoms or prolonged loss of consciousness. Although the duration of loss of consciousness that warrants ER evaluation has not been systematically
evaluated, 1 min is the threshold used by many clinicians to triage to higher levels of
care. "Red flag" signs of cervical injury, more severe intracranial trauma, or skull fracture require further evaluation in an acute care setting. Cervical spine injury should be
suspected based on mechanism of injury (extreme force, axial load), midline neck pain,

tenderness on examination, or motor or sensory changes. More severe intracranial injury should be suspected in the setting of cranial nerve deficits, seizures, deteriorating consciousness, worsening combativeness, persistent or escalating headaches or vomiting, or other focal neurological deficit. Signs of skull fracture include hemotympanum, otorrhea, rhinorrhea, or palpable skull deformity. High-risk mechanisms, such as high-speed impact, fall from significant height, or rotational components are sufficient to warrant higher level evaluation.

Outpatient management: When evaluating an acute SRC in the outpatient setting, a thorough history must be obtained. Mechanism of injury, presence/absence of witness, duration of loss of consciousness, and timing of symptoms onset should be elucidated. A provider should obtain a history of prior concussions, including symptoms and time course for recovery. Relevant comorbidities such as learning disabilities and other cognitive, affective, or behavioral conditions should also be noted. Any pre-injury baseline testing, including computerized neuropsychological screens, should also be reviewed. Standardized symptoms inventories, such as the Acute Concussion Evaluation (ACE) for children or the Rivermead Post Concussion Symptom Questionnaire (RPCSQ), Symptoms Checklist, or Neurobehavioral Symptom Inventory (NSI) for adults, should be completed to monitor evolution of symptoms.

Physical examination of the concussed athlete in the outpatient setting should include assessment of the nervous system, cervical region, vestibular function, oculomotor ability, vision, cognition, and psychological state. Nervous system examination should include testing of cranial nerves, muscle strength, sensation, reflexes, and coordination. Funduscopic examination should be performed to evaluate for papilledema that may indicate increased intracranial pressure (ICP). A neck and shoulder girdle examination should be completed to evaluate for concomitant injuries. Cervical radiculopathy should be suspected with motor or sensory loss in nerve root distribution or positive Spurling's provocative maneuver. Vestibular testing may include Dix-Hallpike maneuver for benign paroxysmal positional vertigo (BPPV) and evaluation for nystagmus. The Balance Error Scoring System (BESS) evaluates postural stability in three different stances on both a hard surface and foam surface. Ocular testing should evaluate alignment, range of motion, smooth pursuit, saccades, vergence (convergence and divergence), vestibular-ocular reflex, and visual motion sensitivity. The King-Devick (K-D) test is a computer-based timed test where patients read numbers across three test cards. The K-D test evaluates visual movement, tracking, attention, and language. Elevated scores have been demonstrated postinjury compared with preinjury baselines and nonconcussed controls. A variety of computerized neuropsychological assessments, such as the Immediate Post-Concussion and Cognitive Testing (ImPACT) and Automated Neuropsychological Assessment Metrics (ANAM), track cognitive recovery after concussion through comparison with baseline testing.

Laboratory studies: The initial laboratory evaluation of the concussed athlete should include checking a serum sodium. Hypo- or hypernatremia can develop in the acute and subacute settings and may require monitoring and correction. Evaluations of blood, saliva, and CSF for novel biomarkers that may aid in the diagnosis of concussion and identification of patients who may have prolonged recovery are being rapidly developed but currently have limited clinical application. There is a single test (Brain Trauma Indicator) approved by the US Food and Drug Administration (FDA); it utilizes UCH–L1 and GFAP, which indicate the presence of intracranial lesions early after concussion and may assist in the decision to obtain CT imaging. The test is not diagnostic of a concussion.

Imaging: Five percent to fifteen percent of mild TBIs (mTBIs) are complicated, meaning that objective changes on imaging exist such as contusion, intraparenchymal hemorrhage, or hematomas in epidural, subdural, or subarachnoid spaces. The Canadian Head CT rules constitute a decision-making tool to aid in the decision to obtain cranial imaging after a concussion. The rule posits that a practitioner should obtain imaging after a suspected concussion if any one of the following is true: the etiology was a dangerous mechanism (i.e., motor-pedestrian accident, motor vehicle accident with ejection, fall from greater than 3 feet or more than 5 stairs), patient is 65 years or older, GCS is less than 15 at 2 h after injury, retrograde amnesia lasts more than 30 min prior to impact, there is suspicion for open or depressed skull fracture including basilar skull fracture (hemotympanum, raccoon eyes, Battle sign), a suspected CSF leak, or two or more episodes of vomiting. MRI and functional imaging are not typically warranted in the acute setting. Axonal injury is likely the pathognomonic lesion underlying concussion, but it is not reliably demonstrated by current clinical imaging modalities. Transcranial Doppler has promise as an adjunctive imaging tool which may risk-stratify patients with the likelihood for neurological deterioration, but its use is not yet common practice.

Questions

1. How would your clinical, laboratory, and radiological findings influence initial management?
2. What parameters are involved in the decision to have this individual return to work?
3. What factors need to be considered before returning this individual to physical activity?

Oral Boards Review: Diagnostic Pearls

- Concussion is a clinical diagnosis: there is no singular physical finding, serum biomarker, or imaging study that is diagnostic of concussion.
  - Concussion should be evaluated in a systematic manner. There are measures such as the SAC and SCAT-5 available for guidance, but no validated cutoff scores for concussion diagnosis.
  - Consider using standardized ocular testing, balance, and computerized cognitive screening as adjuncts to evaluation.
- Concussion diagnosis requires serial examinations as symptoms often evolve with time.
- Orientation after SRC should be evaluated via Maddock's

Questions

- Escalation of care should result from the following: cervical injury, more severe intracranial trauma, or skull fracture or history of a high-risk mechanism.
- Intracranial imaging should be obtained when individuals meet the Canadian Head CT Criteria. These criteria include:
  - Dangerous etiology (i.e., motor-pedestrian accident, motor vehicle accident with ejection, fall from greater than 3 feet or more than 5 stairs)
  - Age greater than 65 years
  - GCS of less than 15 at 2 h after injury
  - Retrograde amnesia lasts more than 30 min prior to impact
  - There is suspicion for open or depressed skull fracture or CSF leak
  - If patient has two or more episodes of vomiting

Decision Making

Disposition: Either inpatient or at-home observation is recommended for at least 24 h after mTBI. Admission for observation should be considered in patients with any of the following: GCS of less than 15, CT abnormalities, neurological deficit, seizures, or persistent vomiting. Admission should also be considered for patients with GCS 15 who do not have a responsible person to monitor them. Alternatively, a head CT can be obtained in patients with GCS of 15 and no options for outpatient observation. A normal head CT has been shown to effectively predict lack of neurological deterioration.

Reassurance and conservative measures are the mainstays of treatment in acute concussion. The majority of symptoms after concussion resolve in 7–10 days with conservative measures (although it is likely that cerebral physiological abnormalities may persist past this time). It is important to communicate with patients the high likelihood of symptom resolution and the typical short time course for recovery. Concussed patients who reported a belief that long-lasting effects were probable after injury have been shown to be more likely to have persisting symptoms at 3 months compared with patients who endorsed likelihood of recovery.

Although the prescription for "relative rest" is not well-defined, a judicious balance between rest and resumption of activity is advantageous. Reasonable restrictions on physical and cognitive activity should be encouraged within the first few days following injury. Typically, activity that does not provoke or exacerbate symptoms is permitted. Optional cognitive stressors such as video games or large social gatherings may be limited in the acute period. Restrictions should be individualized to the patient's severity, symptoms, and responsibilities. The degree and duration of relative rest should be frequently reassessed. In the pediatric and adolescent population, prolonged rest or complete rest with strict limitations from school can be associated with development of prolonged postconcussive symptoms. Education should be provided regarding sleep hygiene and adequate hydration and nutrition in the acute period.

Acutely, pharmacologic intervention should target symptom management. Over-the-counter analgesics such as acetaminophen or nonsteroidal anti-inflammatory drugs may be used for tension headache management. Headaches with a significant migraine component may respond to a short-duration therapy with triptan medications. Substances that may adversely affect cognition such as opioids, muscle relaxants, alcohol, marijuana, and illicit drugs should be avoided.

Return to school and work protocols should be individualized to the patient's symptoms and functional impairments. For children, a formal 504 educational plan can be arranged for short-term accommodations. Return to learning should take place in a staged fashion. Initially, children should be encouraged to participate in typical, daily activities around the home. If asymptomatic, they may progress to light cognitive activities such as reading or homework outside of the classroom. Following, they can return to school part-time, starting with 1–3 h and extending length of school day to a full day. When returning to the classroom, students may need accommodations such as increased breaks during the day, shorter assignments, repetition of material, and later start times. Similarly, adults may need work accommodations including gradual extension of work hours, frequent rest breaks, limited computer use, and extensions on assignments.

A return to sport protocol should be initiated once a return to learn/work protocol has been completed and the individual is tolerating a full school or work day. Individuals progress through each of the six steps in the return-to-play protocol and require a minimum of 24 h at each stage; therefore, it should take a minimum of 1 week to progress through the entire protocol. The initial stage of any return-to-play protocol involves tolerating daily activities without exacerbation of symptoms. Individuals should progress through light aerobic exercise, sport-specific exercise, noncontact drill, and full contact practice before returning to sport. During progression, if any concussion-related symptoms recur, the individual should continue at the previous, asymptomatic level and reattempt progression after another 24 h free of symptoms.

Questions

1. Which population would require more monitoring for delayed intracranial pathology?
2. What is the most common type of intracranial process requiring surgical intervention that occurs after concussion?

Surgical Procedure

Surgery is rarely indicated in the setting of concussion, except in the case of delayed subdural hematoma (SDH) or other intracranial bleed. With a history of blunt trauma, about 8% of patient will require neurosurgical intervention. Of patients requiring intervention, isolated epidural hemorrhage or isolated subdural hemorrhage were most frequently associated with need for neurosurgical procedure. Of patients with SDH, older patients required surgery more often than younger patients.

Oral Boards Review: Management Pearls

- Relative rest should involve a balance of resumption of activities and rest. The timing and dosage of rest is being elucidated.

- Return to work should be individualized according to occupational safety and critical work activities.
- Return to play should follow a stepwise protocol with a minimum of 7 days out of contact sports.
- Coexisting medical, psychological, and social factors should be considered in the management of concussion.

Pivot Points

- If a patient has neurological deterioration, the patient needs re-evaluation and possibly reimaging to evaluate for progressive intracranial process that may require surgical intervention.
- Persistent symptoms should be managed by a multidisciplinary team.

Aftercare

The natural history of concussion depends on both premorbid and injury-related factors. For most, symptoms are most severe within the first 24–72 h and may include a variety of somatic, affective, and cognitive symptoms. These acute symptoms typically dissipate within a week after injury. A majority of patients have improved and have returned to normal activity by 4 weeks, with 85–90% of patients having full resolution by 3 months.

Complications and Management

Neurological deterioration following an mTBI suggests an evolving intracranial process, such as hematoma, and should be evaluated and managed as described elsewhere in this book. SDH may present in the acute, subacute, or chronic phase and should be considered with delayed deterioration, especially in the elderly.

Second-impact syndrome (SIS) is a devastating and possibly lethal complication that occurs when an individual experiences a second concussion while still symptomatic from a prior concussion. Disrupted autoregulation of cerebral blood flow may result in diffuse and rapid cerebral swelling leading to increased ICP and herniation, ultimately resulting in coma or death. There is no specific management for this condition other than addressing increased ICP in a timely manner. It is imperative to prevent a second head injury while an individual is still recovering from an initial mTBI to mitigate risk of SIS.

Chronic postconcussive syndrome (PCS) describes a constellation of symptoms persisting beyond 3 months after injury. Reports of incidence of chronic PCS range from 5% to 15% at 1 year post mTBI. Risk factors for prolonged symptoms include female gender, lower initial GCS, complicated mTBI, severity of initial symptoms, history of head injury, premorbid history of neurological disease or psychiatric disease, pending litigation, and older age. The most commonly reported symptoms include persistent headache, fatigue, sleep disturbance, dizziness, neck pain, and cognitive dysfunction. Self-report scales, such as the Post-Concussive Symptom Scale-Revised

(PCSS-R) and the Rivermead Post-Concussion Symptom Questionnaire, may be used to track symptom evolution over time. Diagnostic evaluation of patients with chronic PCS may include serum screens of the hypothalamic-pituitary axis, although this is not yet standard of care. Individuals with persistent, functionally limiting symptoms may benefit from MRI to exclude other pathology. There are currently no clinical guidelines to support or refute use of functional neuroimaging in the subacute or chronic phases of mTBI. Neuropsychological evaluation may be needed for patients with significant behavioral or cognitive complaints and can be additionally useful in individuals with suspected comorbid psychological illness and pain syndromes. Advanced vestibular testing should be sought out in patients with vertigo with accompanying postural instability, auditory symptoms, or nystagmus. Advanced ocular evaluation should be sought out in patients with signs of ocular dysmotility or change in visual acuity.

Treatment of chronic postconcussive syndrome is aimed at symptom relief and improved function and often involves multidisciplinary care. Patients with chronic postconcussive syndrome benefit from education and continued management of premorbid issues. Posttraumatic headache (PTH) is common after concussion. To guide management, providers should determine headache type such as migraine, tension, cervicogenic, temporomandibular-joint related, intracranial hypotension, or occipital neuralgia. Tension-type PTH can be managed with conservative measures such as adequate hydration, sufficient sleep, nonsteroidal anti-inflammatory drugs, and relative rest. Migraine-type PTH may response to triptan medications for abortive treatment in conjunction with tricyclic antidepressants or beta-blockers for preventative management. Providers should address comorbid conditions that may contribute to headaches, such as sleep disturbance, mood disturbance, or ocular dysfunction.

Cervical pathology after concussion may contribute to local or referred pain, headaches, and balance deficits. After excluding skeletal fractures, vascular injury, and neurological compromise, treatment options for biomechanical cervical pathology may include manual therapy, mobilization, stretching, application of modalities, acupuncture, or injections.

Dizziness and balance impairment after concussion has a broad differential including benign paroxysmal positional vertigo, labyrinthine concussion, perilymphatic fistula, direct trauma to vestibular organs, vertebral artery dissection, epileptic vertigo, vestibular migraine, and panic attack. A comprehensive vestibular rehabilitation program may include therapy for adaptation and compensation, otolaryngology evaluation and management, and ocular evaluation and management.

Physical, mental, and cognitive fatigue in postconcussive syndrome is multifactorial. Evaluation for psychiatric, cardiovascular, sleep-related, endocrine-related, infectious, and medication effects should be completed and addressed. Nonpharmacological management includes initiation of routine exercise and education on energy conservation strategies. Pharmacologic management is reserved for chronic cases and, currently, has limited evidence. Treatment options may include modafinil, donepezil, or methylphenidate.

Postconcussive cognitive dysfunction most often involves deficits in attention, concentration, processing speed, or memory. Neuropsychological testing can help identify specific deficits that may be targets for cognitive therapy, accommodations, or pharmacologic interventions.

Oral Boards Review: Complication Pearls

- SIS may result when an individual sustains a concussion while still symptomatic from an initial concussion. Disrupted cerebral blood flow is thought to underlie SIS and may lead to increased ICP requiring surgical management.
- Persistent concussion symptoms may prompt further imaging, such as MRI, to evaluate for coexisting conditions.
- Neuropsychological evaluation with a skilled examiner may help guide therapeutic strategies and return to activity.
- Headache is the most common physical complaint after concussion. There should be targeted management of headaches after concussion to prevent development of chronic headaches.
- Fatigue is often multifactorial. Management includes optimization of sleep, mood, pain syndromes, and potential endocrine abnormalities.

Evidence and Outcomes

The long-term implications of repetitive head trauma are still being elucidated. There is inconsistent evidence that repetitive concussions may cause cumulative psychological, cognitive, and motor effects. Limited studies have shown increased rates of depression, suicidality, personality change, dementia, and parkinsonism after repetitive trauma. Protracted or increased severity of symptoms may also be seen with repetitive trauma. The mechanism of long-term cognitive effects of repetitive mTBI is still unknown, but it has been suggested that brain trauma may cause a neuroinflammatory response and/or activate pathologic mechanisms similar to those associated with Alzheimer's disease. The role of repetitive subconcussive blows to development of long-term sequelae is also undetermined.

Currently, there are no clinical criteria for diagnosis of *chronic traumatic encephalopathy*. The degree, type, and number of cerebral traumas required to cause CTE is also unknown. There have been reports of CTE following multiple sports concussions, single TBI, or multiple military mTBIs. Ultimately, a causal mechanistic link between trauma and CTE is yet to be described.

Further Reading

Borg J, Holm L, Cassidy JD, et al. Diagnostic procedures in mild traumatic brain injury: Results of the WHO Collaborating Task Force on Mild Traumatic Brain Injury. *J Rehabil Med.* 2004;61.

Echemendia RJ, Meeuwisse W, McCrory P, et al. The Sport Concussion Assessment Tool 5th Edition (SCAT5): Background and rationale. *Br J Sports Med.* 2017;51:848–850.

Feddermann-Demont N, Echemendia RJ, Schneider KJ, et al. What domains of clinical function should be assessed after sport-related concussion? A systematic review. *Br J Sports Med.* 2017; 51(11):903–918.

Gibson S, Nigrovic LE, O'Brien M, Meehan WP 3rd. The effect of recommending cognitive rest on recovery from sport-related concussion. *Brain Inj.* 2013;27:839.

Giza CC, Kuthcer JD, Ashwal S, et al. Summary of evidence-based guideline update: Evaluation and management of concussion in sports: Report of the Guideline Development Subcommittee of the American Academy of Neurology. *Neurology.* 2013;80: 2250

Halstead ME, et al. Returning to learning following a concussion. *Pediatrics.* 2013;132(5): 948–57.

Jagoda AS, Bazarian JJ, Bruns JJ, et al. Clinical policy: Neuroimaging and decision making in adult mild traumatic brain injury in the acute setting. *Ann Emerg Med.* 2008;52:714–748

McCrory P, Meeuwisse W, Dvořák J, et al. Consensus statement on concussion in sport-the 5(th) international conference on concussion in sport held in Berlin, October 2016. *Br J Sports Med.* 2017;51(11):838–847.

Ponsford J, Willmott C, Rothwell A, et al. Impact of early intervention on outcome following mild head injury in adults. *J Neurol Neurosurg Psychiatry* 2002;73:330.

Calvarial Vault Fractures

Philip A. Villanueva and Erin Graves

10

Case Presentation

A 24-year-old man is brought to the trauma center, having been struck with an unknown object over his right temporal region. There is scalp swelling but no laceration. By report, he did not lose consciousness. His Glasgow Coma Score (GCS) is 14 (4E, 4V [disoriented to time], 6M). Aside from swelling and tenderness in the right temporal area and disorientation, his examination is intact. Head and neck CT scans are ordered. While awaiting these, the patient becomes more lethargic and disoriented (GCS 11 [3,3,5])

Questions

1. What is the likely diagnosis?
2. What is the appropriate imaging study?
3. What is the proper timing of the workup?

Assessment and Planning

The consulting neurosurgeon suspects a temporal bone fracture with underlying intracranial hematoma. Other diagnoses include diffuse brain swelling, a subclinical seizure with a postictal state, or a major concussion. The location and mechanism places the fracture diagnosis high on the differential list. Prior to the advent of CT scanning, plain skull x-rays were the routine diagnostic modality. CT scanning allows the clinician to both diagnose accurately as well as plan any surgical intervention.

Oral Boards Review: Diagnostic Pearls

- Calvarial or vault fractures may be considered in several ways:
  - Closed versus open fractures. With closed fractures, the galea over the fracture is intact. With open fractures the galea is torn and the fracture exposed. In addition to the concern for scalp bleeding due to galeal vessel injury, the exposure of the fracture may result in exposure of the intracranial contents beneath the fracture, thus increasing the risk of infection (Figure. 10.1).
  - Linear versus comminuted versus depressed fractures. Linear fractures, as the name implies, are generally nonbranching, generally do not cross suture

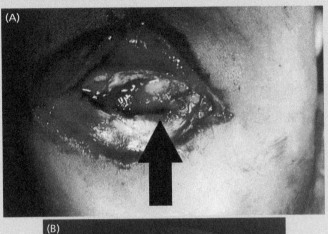

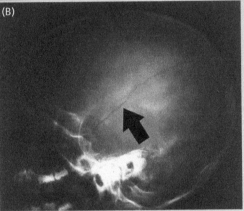

Figure 10.1 (A) Open depressed calvarial fracture (arrow) with exposed dura. (B) Linear, non-depressed calvarial fracture (arrow).

lines, and bone on both sides of the fracture remains co-planar (Figure 10.2). Depressed fractures refer to a difference in height between the fracture plates (Figure 10.3A,B). Comminuted fractures are characterized by fragmentation of the bone plates, and these fragments may be co-planar or depressed (Figure 10.4).

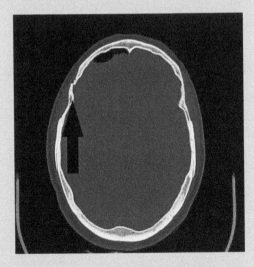

Figure 10.2 Closed depressed calvarial fracture (arrow).

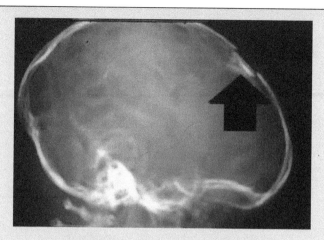

Figure 10.3 Open, comminuted calvarial fracture (arrow).

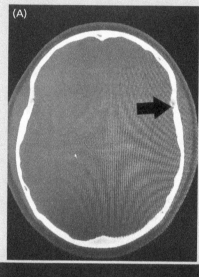

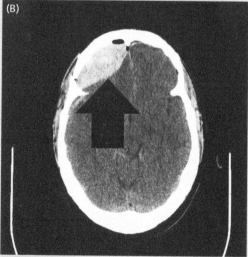

Figure 10.4 (A) "Green-stick" fracture overlying middle meningeal artery (arrow). (B) Depressed fracture causing epidural hematoma due to laceration of middle meningeal artery (arrow). (C) Epidural hematoma (arrow) caused by tear of transverse sinus by occipital fracture.

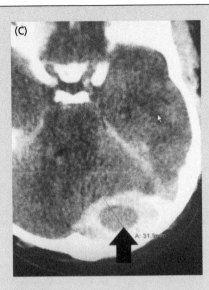

Figure 10.4 (A) (Continued)

- Diagnosis is usually made via CT scan, although, in the case of open fractures, the pathology may be seen and/or palpated (very carefully!).

Not all calvarial fractures may be easily seen on CT. The clinician must differentiate between the fracture and normal findings such as vascular markings and suture lines. Careful viewing of the axial views may reveal a splitting of the bone or a "green-stick" (Figure 10.5) type fracture. In addition, CT will also reveal a secondary injury to the underlying brain, such as a contusion or frank hematoma (Figure 10.6).

In the case of depressed and/or comminuted fracture, the offending bone may be identified more clearly for surgical elevation/removal. The CT may also reveal intracranial air, indicating a concomitant or contiguous skull base fracture. Also of value with CT scanning is the assessment of fractures involving cranial air sinuses. Presence of an underlying hematoma and/or pneumocephalus may require surgical intervention.

On occasion, if there is no need for acute surgical intervention, 3-D CT reconstruction may be of value in assessing bone fragments, and CT angiography may be helpful in determining the presence of a vascular injury. This is frequently encountered when fracture lines or comminuted bone fragments involve arterial canals or major dural venous sinuses.

In the case of the patient presented here, CT scanning revealed a linear right temporal fracture crossing the middle meningeal artery and resulting in an epidural hematoma (Figure 10.7).

Questions

1. How do imaging findings influence possible surgical planning?
2. What is the time frame for intervention in this patient?
3. If a CT angiogram is not performed, what factors must be taken into consideration?

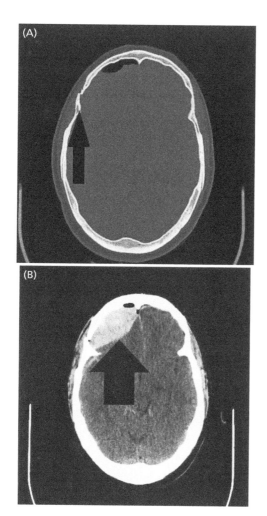

Figure 10.5 (A) Linear calvarial fracture overlying right middle meningeal artery (arrow). (B) Resultant epidural hematoma due to laceration of middle meningeal artery.

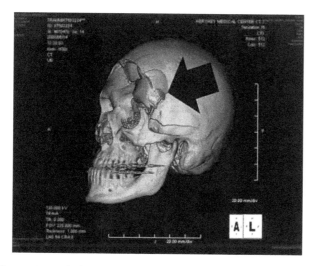

Figure 10.6 Comminuted/depressed calvarial and basilar fracture involving left orbit.

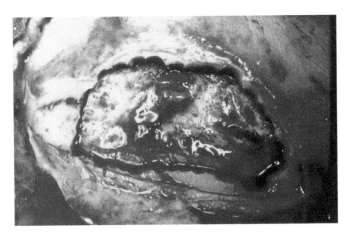

Figure 10.7 Craniectomy for open, depressed, comminuted calvarial fracture.

Decision Making

A simple linear, nondepressed, closed fracture requires no special treatment after CT scanning other than cleansing and closure of any associated scalp wound(s). If the galea is torn over a linear fracture, broad-spectrum oral antibiotics may be given for a 7-day period at the clinician's discretion. If diffuse intracranial air seen, the likelihood of a basilar fracture is high and attention must be directed to identifying this. Patients with uncomplicated linear fractures may incur a concussion requiring follow-up treatment.

In the case of a hematoma, the Guidelines are helpful in determining the need for operative intervention. If the fracture is closed and either comminuted or significantly depressed (greater than the thickness of the adjacent skull), surgical intervention is undertaken to elevate and internally fix with titanium plating the depressed fracture plates.

If the fracture is noted to be depressed/comminuted and open, consideration must be given to performing a craniectomy if there is gross contamination (soil, foreign body, in-driven hair). Otherwise the surgeon may opt to replace the larger bone fragments. Smaller fragments, if contaminated, may become foci for infection and, even if not contaminated, may undergo bone resorption resulting in a bony gap.

Questions

1. How does a scalp laceration affect the skin incision?
2. What are the options for bony reconstruction after fracture?

Surgical Procedure

Surgical repair of skull fractures is usually performed under general anesthesia, with two peripheral IVs and an arterial line in place. Bladder catheterization is usually not needed unless the case is expected to last more than 2 h or the patient's volume status is critical. The patient is usually supine (unless prone for an occipital lesion) and the head is placed on a rest of the surgeon's choice. Usually pin fixation is not needed unless the patient is prone or in the lateral position. The location of the fracture dictates the incision, but if there is an attendant hematoma, wider rather than narrower exposure should be the rule. If there is an overlying laceration, the surgeon may opt to extend the laceration in a "Lazy-S" manner, or incorporate the laceration into the incision line, or include it within the scalp flap. Dural bleeding is controlled with bipolar cautery, and dural edges may be tacked up to prevent extradural dissection.

If the dura is penetrated by bone fragments, they should be removed carefully with the most in-driven fragments being removed last. Meticulous parenchymal hemostasis is maintained throughout. Dural tears are traditionally repaired in a watertight manner, although some surgeons utilize a dural substitute placed over the dura.

As noted previously, clean bony defects may be covered with a titanium plate or mesh and possibly a layer of bone cement or methylmethacrylate. Antibiotic irrigation is used throughout, and, in the case of open wounds, culturing the wound prior to antibiotic irrigation may help in identifying an infectious agent postoperatively. A subgaleal drain is often placed as the scalp may be bruised or traumatized from the initial injury. The scalp is closed in layers and a sterile dressing placed. Postoperative CT scanning is obtained to assess the operative site as well as other areas where delayed bleeding or swelling may have occurred. Generally the patient is extubated in the operating room or ICU depending on the preoperative GCS, intraoperative findings, and emergence from anesthesia.

Oral Boards Review: Management Pearls

- The presence of a skull fracture even in a patient with a "normal" neurological exam increases the chance of an intracranial hematoma.
- The elderly patient is prone to backward falls with concomitant fractures involving the torcula and the transverse sinuses (Figure 10.6). Because these are venous structures, bleeding may be significantly slower than from arterial sources and develop later. This population is also frequently on anticoagulant therapy. Hence repeat CT scanning should be performed approximately 4–6 h after the initial scan or if there is neurological decline. Subsequent studies may be obtained 12 and 24 h following the initial study.

Pivot Points

- If there is unexpected swelling during a fracture repair, or if there is uncertainty as to the presence of contamination, rather than place a construct in a contaminated field, default to the adage, "when in doubt, leave it out" and perform a craniectomy.
- If the fracture is associated with an epidural hematoma which is resected, anticonvulsant therapy is usually not continued past a week. Likewise, if there is traumatic subarachnoid bleeding, it is also not continued past 7 days. Dural and cortical lacerations are associated with delayed seizures, and patients should be warned of that possibility with instructions regarding further follow-up care.

Aftercare

In the case of the uncomplicated, simple linear fracture, management is very similar to that of a moderate to severe concussion; overnight observation, no anticonvulsants, avoidance of narcotic analgesics, and preferential therapy with nonsteroidal anti-inflammatory medications.

In the case of the patient who has undergone surgery, initial analgesia may be achieved with narcotics but a rapid transition to nonsteroidals is usually made. Some patients may have postoperative pain due to dural irritation. In this situation, valproic acid 500–1,500 mg/d may be helpful. Patients are mobilized as rapidly as practicable, and evaluations by rehabilitation services are made to determine if post-acute discharge rehabilitation is indicated. Unless otherwise indicated, a 1-month postoperative CT is obtained; however, earlier and later studies may be performed depending on the severity of the injury.

Complications and Management

The most common complication of calvarial fractures is delayed bleeding. This is most frequently seen among patients who have a primary coagulation disorder or are on anticoagulants. Another group, usually a younger age group, are those patients with active hematopoiesis in their cranial bones. Diploic bleeding in this group may well be delayed and insidious. Worsening headache after the primary injury, with or without delayed neurological deficits, should usually prompt the clinician to repeat imaging. "Growing" fractures, relatively common in the pediatric population, also occur in the adolescent population. Nonetheless, a progressively expanding and pulsatile mass in the area of the linear fracture should also be investigated with CT imaging. Infection following surgical repair ranges from 5% to up to 25% (reflecting contaminated cases). Generally, a waiting period of approximately 6 months is allowed to expire before reconstruction of a contaminated cranial defect is undertaken, with sedimentation rate (ESR) and c-reactive protein (CRP) levels sent prior to admissions for the procedures. For "clean" cases, a waiting period of 1–3 months (or until any brain swelling subsides) is common.

Oral Boards Review: Complications Pearls

- A progressively expanding, pulsatile mass in the area of a fracture should be investigated with imaging to evaluate for a "growing fracture."
- The waiting period of at least 6 months or so is customary after a contaminated or infected procedure to ensure that the cranioplasty is being placed in a clean field.

Evidence and Outcome

Much of the discussion regarding calvarial fractures revolves around management of the intracranial sequelae of the trauma: bleed, infection, posttraumatic epilepsy. The uncomplicated injuries are usually self-limited problems. As for managing the secondary problems, various guidelines for management of traumatic brain injury are available.

Further Reading

Mendelow AD, Campbell D, Tsementzis SA, et al. Prophylactic antimicrobial management of compound depressed skull fracture. *JR Coll Surg Edinb.* 1983;28(2):80–83.

Servadei F, Ciucci G, Pagano F, et al. Skull fracture as a risk factor of intracranial complications in minor head injuries: A prospective CT study in a series of 98 adult patients. *J Neurol Neurosurg Psychiatry.* 1988;51(4):526–528.

Valadka AB. Injury to cranium. In Moore F, Mattox K, eds. *Trauma.* New York: McGraw Hill; 2008:385–406.

Traumatic Anterior Cranial Fossa CSF Leaks

Omaditya Khanna, Tomas Garzon-Muvdi, Hermes Garcia,
Richard F. Schmidt, James J. Evans, and Christopher J. Farrell

Case Presentation

A 20-year-old female pedestrian was brought to the emergency department by ambulance after being struck by a motor vehicle. She was intubated in the field and immobilized in a rigid cervical collar. Upon arrival in the trauma bay, the patient did not follow commands or open her eyes to stimuli, but she moved all of her extremities spontaneously and symmetrically (Glasgow Coma Scale [GCS] score of 7T). There was soft tissue swelling of the face with serosanguineous discharge emanating from the patient's nares and crusted blood visible in the bilateral external auditory canals. Cranial nerve examination demonstrated normal pupillary constriction along with preserved gag and corneal reflexes. No scalp lacerations or palpable cranial deformities were noted on initial inspection.

Questions

1. In addition to a traumatic brain injury, what other diagnoses are highly suspected?
2. What imaging studies are indicated for the initial evaluation of this patient?
3. What lab tests and imaging modalities are available to assist in the diagnosis of traumatic CSF leaks?
4. What special precautions should be taken in this patient?

Assessment and Planning

Based on the arrival GCS, physical examination, and mechanism of injury, a severe traumatic brain injury with likely basilar skull base fracture and traumatic CSF was highly suspected. Hemotympanum is often indicative of a basilar skull fracture and may appear within hours of the traumatic injury. Bilateral periorbital ecchymoses ("raccoon eyes") and mastoid ecchymoses ("Battle's sign") are also predictive of a basilar skull fracture but typically occur in a delayed fashion 1–3 days after the injury. Due to the concern for a basilar skull fracture, a CT scan of the head along with high-resolution CT scans of the skull base and facial bones were obtained. The CT showed bilateral inferior frontal lobe hemorrhagic contusions, a displaced right frontal calvarial fracture, and bilateral ethmoid roof fractures (Figure 11.1). The right frontal fracture was noted to extend through both the anterior and posterior tables of the frontal sinus and into the roof of the right orbit.

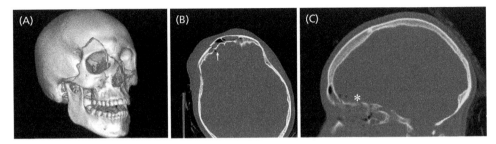

Figure 11.1 (A) 3D high-resolution CT reconstruction demonstrating a right frontal bone fracture with extension through the orbital roof and anterior table of frontal sinus. (B) Axial CT showing displaced anterior and posterior table (*arrow*) fractures of the frontal sinus with pneumocephalus. (C) Sagittal CT reconstruction demonstrating frontal sinus and ethmoidal roof fractures (★).

Scattered areas of pneumocephalus were noted posterior to the frontal sinus fracture and above the ethmoidal roof fractures.

Traumatic CSF leaks are reported in 10–30% of skull base fractures. The majority of these leaks present within the first 48 h of the traumatic insult, although occasionally traumatic CSF leaks may present in a delayed fashion weeks or months following the initial trauma.[1] The most common fracture sites leading to CSF leakage are injury to the frontal sinus (31%), sphenoid sinus (11–31%), ethmoid sinuses (15–19%), and the cribriform plate (6%).[2]

The diagnosis of CSF leak is made through observation of clear drainage emanating from the nose or ears, which is often reproducible via dependent positioning by sitting the patient up and flexing their neck forward after a period of recumbency (reservoir sign). Fluid discharge from the nose and ear can be further evaluated via a "target sign" or "halo ring" seen on filter paper. However, signs of CSF leak may be more difficult to discern in the posttraumatic setting, and further testing may be required to confirm the diagnosis.

β2-transferrin (β2Tr) is a protein that is found in the CSF, perilymph, and aqueous humor, but not in nasal secretions. Laboratory confirmation of β2Tr presence in nasal drainage specimens is highly sensitive (99%) and specific (97%) for diagnosing CSF leaks. Although only a small amount of fluid is necessary for laboratory evaluation, collection of an adequate specimen can be difficult in slow, intermittent leaks. β-trace protein (βTP) is another protein that is present at a higher concentration in CSF compared to plasma, and it has both a high positive and negative predictive value (97% and 100%, respectively). Although βTP is less expensive and has a shorter processing time (~30 min) than β2Tr, it is not available at many institutions and is not suitable for use in patients with proven or suspected meningitis.[3]

There are various imaging modalities available for the evaluation of patients with craniofacial trauma and for preoperative planning in patients who require surgical intervention for reconstruction and repair of CSF fistulae. A high-resolution CT (HRCT) with 1–2 mm sections and axial, coronal, and sagittal reconstructions is usually the first study performed as it is very sensitive for the detection of fractures and localization of potential CSF leakage sites.[4] CT is less accurate in detecting thin nondisplaced fractures, and nonpathologic areas of thin or absent portions of the bony skull base may sometimes be misinterpreted as a fracture.

Adjunctive imaging modalities may be necessary in patients with clinically apparent CSF leakage and multiple skull base fractures in order to correctly determine the actual site of CSF leakage. Alternatively, these imaging studies may be indicated in patients with clinically suspected but unconfirmed CSF leakage in order to appropriately establish the diagnosis. CT cisternography requires intrathecal administration of a radiopaque contrast dye such as metrizamide, iohexol, or iopamidol and has been shown to detect 80% of CSF fistulae. This study is most useful for identifying anterior cranial fossa leaks into the nasal sinuses where pooling of the contrast can be visualized. MR cisternography is a noninvasive method that uses T2-weighted fat suppression images and phase reversal to identify areas of CSF accumulation. MR cisternography is also very helpful in imaging soft tissue structures and identifying meningo-encephaloceles; however, this imaging modality is unable to establish whether there is an active leak and does not evaluate bony anatomy well. When used in combination, CT and MR imaging results can identify the site of CSF leakage in 90% of cases.[5]

Oral Boards Review: Diagnostic Pearls

- β_2Tr is a protein that is found in the CSF and not in nasal secretions; it has a high sensitivity (99%) and specificity (97%) for diagnosing CSF leaks.
- A HRCT of the skull base is the initial imaging modality used to evaluate for cranial and facial bone fractures that may be responsible for CSF leakage.
- CT cisternography (using an intrathecal contrast dye) and MR cisternography are adjunctive imaging modalities that can be used to confirm the presence of a CSF leak and identify the site of leakage.

Questions

1. How long can one try nonsurgical measures or CSF diversion before proceeding to surgery?
2. What are the other indications for surgery?
3. Is there a role for nonoperative treatment of delayed CSF leaks?

Decision Making

Traumatic CSF leaks may be treated conservatively or via surgical repair. Nonsurgical management of CSF leaks includes bed rest with head-of-bed elevation, sinus precautions (no nose blowing, sneezing, or Valsalva maneuvers), and carbonic anhydrase inhibitors to lower intracranial pressure (ICP) and facilitate dural healing. The majority (50–85%) of traumatic CSF leaks resolve spontaneously and do not require surgical intervention.[6] In patients with persistent leakage or in those for whom healing is unlikely to occur (penetrating trauma, large bony defects, elevated ICP), additional treatment may be necessary to prevent complications such as meningitis or pneumocephalus. CSF diversion maneuvers such as serial lumbar punctures or extended lumbar drainage can help augment spontaneous resolution by reducing active CSF flow through the leak. External ventricular drain placement may also be used to resolve CSF fistulae as well as to monitor ICP in patients with a poor neurological exam. The length of time of conservative management is controversial, but the risk of meningitis increases from 5% to 11% at the end of 7 days to 55–88% in patients with persistent CSF leakage lasting beyond 1 week.[7] Additionally, conservative management is usually reserved for patients who do not require surgical intervention for correction of a fracture or other intracranial injury.

Surgical intervention for traumatic CSF leakage may be performed in either an early or delayed fashion and using either an open transcranial or endoscopic endonasal approach. Due to the high rate of spontaneous resolution of CSF fistulae with conservative measures, early surgical repair within the first several days after the trauma is usually reserved for patients with extenuating circumstances. Patients with intracerebral hematomas requiring evacuation or with penetrating injury may benefit from simultaneous repair of the CSF leakage site if accessible. Similarly, if surgical reconstruction of the facial bones or calvarium is necessary, it may be appropriate to repair the CSF fistula at the time of intervention. Traumatic injuries resulting in large bony skull base defects (>1 cm) or brain herniation are also unlikely to heal with conservative measures and typically require surgical intervention in the early setting. Fractures associated with compressive amounts of pneumocephalus (tension pneumocephalus) or progressively worsening pneumocephalus should be treated with early surgical repair to prevent further complications. Delayed surgery is indicated for patients who fail conservative management or with significant traumatic brain injury and elevated ICP for whom earlier intervention may result in further neurological injury. Additionally, surgery is typically delayed in patients who develop meningitis until their encephalopathy has resolved and they demonstrate a positive laboratory response to antibiotic therapy. Patients who present with a delayed (>1 week) CSF leak after trauma have a low likelihood of spontaneous resolution if treated via conservative measures, and these patients have a very high incidence of developing meningitis.[8] Surgical repair of CSF leak decreases the overall risk of developing meningitis from 30% to 4% in the acute setting with an appreciable 10-year reduction from 85% to 7%.[9]

Surgical repair of traumatic anterior cranial fossa CSF leaks can be achieved via an open transcranial or endoscopic endonasal approach. Traditionally, the open transcranial approach has been favored due to its widespread familiarity among neurosurgeons and ability to access the entire anterior cranial fossa and perform primary repair of dural defects. However, based on the excellent results achieved using the endoscopic endonasal approach for closure of spontaneous CSF leaks, this approach has been increasingly applied in the traumatic setting. Fractures of the frontal sinus with displacement of the posterior table of the frontal sinus are usually most appropriately managed with an open approach. Typically utilizing a bicoronal incision with bilateral anterior craniotomy, this approach facilitates exenteration of the frontal sinus mucosa and complete sinus obliteration to prevent mucocele formation, along with removal of the disrupted posterior wall (cranialization) and dural reconstruction. Patients who require open surgical repair for fixation of facial or calvarial fractures may also be appropriate for simultaneous repair of the CSF fistula site. In patients with multiple skull base fractures and potential sites of CSF leakage, the open transcranial approach provides access to the entirety of the anterior cranial fossa with the ability to directly visualize and repair areas of dural incompetence and achieve a wide skull base repair with a vascularized pericranial flap. Complications of this approach include frontal lobe contusions and hemorrhage from brain retraction, seizures, and anosmia related to injury to the olfactory fossa from extradural dissection.

Overall, open surgery is associated with higher morbidity compared to the less invasive endoscopic endonasal approach, and the endoscopic approach is rapidly becoming the preferred approach for small- to moderate-sized anterior cranial fossa defects involving the cribriform, ethmoid, and sphenoid sinus locations. Large series of endoscopic CSF leak repair have reported success rates of up to 98% with complication rates of only 1–2.5%.[2,10,11] Endoscopic repair involves visualization of the site of CSF leakage, removal of the surrounding mucosa, and multilayered repair of the dural defect using onlay or inlay graft materials. Successful repair of CSF leaks using a variety of autologous and allograft materials has been reported, including fascia lata, temporalis fascia, mucosal grafts, and synthetic dural substitutes. Larger defects may require an additional layer of repair with either a vascularized nasoseptal or turbinate flap. Early endoscopic repair is frequently difficult in patients with associated facial injuries due to concomitant soft tissue and sinus injuries that make access and visualization more difficult. Delayed intervention once the swelling has resolved is typically more appropriate if there is conservative management failure. Intrathecal fluorescein may also be used as an adjunct to the endonasal approach for intraoperative localization of the site of CSF leakage. The fluorescein is administered via lumbar puncture or through a lumbar drain with reported rare complications including allergic reactions, seizures, headaches, and pulmonary edema.[12] While the endoscopic endonasal approach is not typically indicated for posterior table frontal sinus fractures, endoscopic relief of frontal sinus outflow obstruction or drainage of delayed mucoceles may be appropriate.

Questions

1. What are the relative indications for open versus endoscopic surgery?
2. If the leak is not localized on CT or MR imaging, what are other diagnostic tests that might locate it?

Surgical Procedure

The patient was diagnosed with a severe traumatic brain injury and multiple anterior cranial fossa fractures and potential sites of CSF leakage. Given her poor neurological exam, a right frontal external ventriculostomy was placed to manage her elevated ICP and provide CSF diversion. The patient was evaluated by a multidisciplinary team including neurosurgery, otolaryngology, and ophthalmology, and a combined treatment plan was formulated. Due to the patient's multiple fractures, including a displaced posterior table frontal sinus fracture and need for surgical stabilization of her facial fractures, the decision was made to proceed with open transcranial repair once her ICP had normalized. A bicoronal incision was performed and a wide vascularized pericranial flap harvested. A bifrontal craniotomy flap was turned, extending the bony

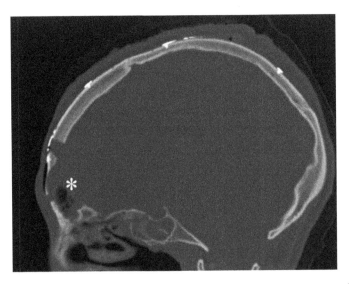

Figure 11.2 Postoperative sagittal CT reconstruction demonstrating cranialization of the frontal sinus with removal of the posterior table of frontal sinus (★) and nasofrontal duct obliteration.

removal to the lateral aspects of the frontal sinus. The frontal lobe dura was carefully separated from the posterior wall of the frontal sinus and the dura of the anterior cranial fossa elevated to expose the bilateral ethmoidal roof fractures. CSF drainage via the external ventriculostomy and diuretic administration were utilized for brain relaxation and to minimize retraction. Areas of dural injury adjacent to the fracture sites were identified and primarily repaired. The posterior wall of the frontal sinus was removed (Figure 11.2) and the mucosa of the frontal sinus and nasal frontal recesses fully removed. The bony margins of the frontal sinus were then drilled with a diamond bit burr to remove any invaginations of mucosa within the bone and prevent delayed mucocele formation. Once the sinus had been fully exenterated, the nasofrontal out-flow tracts were obstructed with temporalis fascia, although a variety of alternative materials may also be used for sinus obliteration including adipose tissue, muscle, pericranium, and bone. The vascularized pericranial flap was then rotated over the frontal sinus and used to cover the ethmoidal roof fractures and prevent persistent CSF leakage. The bone flap was then replaced, leaving a sufficient bony margin to prevent vascular compromise of the pericranial flap. The orbital fracture was also realigned for stabilization and improved cosmesis.

Oral Boards Review: Management Pearls

- Relative indications for surgery for traumatic CSF fistulae:
  - Associated intracranial injuries (intracranial hemorrhage, penetrating injury with foreign body, depressed skull fracture) that require surgical intervention
  - Fractures with a large bony defect (>1 cm) or presence of a meningoencephalocele that may prevent fracture healing

- Patients presenting with delayed posttraumatic CSF leakage (>1 week)
- Persistent CSF leakage (>7 days) refractory to conservative measures

---

Pivot Points

- While most CSF leaks resolve without surgery, patients with leaks lasting longer than 1 week are surgical candidates.
- Endoscopic and open repair are both viable surgical treatments. Relative indications for open repair include the presence of a displaced posterior frontal sinus wall, large or multiple skull base fractures, and the presence of other conditions requiring surgery (e.g., other fractures, hematomas).
- A patient with elevated ICP or meningitis is usually treated surgically after these conditions have resolved.

Aftercare

Patients who undergo endoscopic endonasal procedures should be placed on strict sinus precautions, including head-of-bed elevation (>30 degrees), no nose blowing/sneezing/Valsalva maneuvers, and avoidance of placement of nasogastric tubes without direct visualization. Endoscopic debridement of the nasal sinuses is typically recommended in the postoperative period to prevent synechiae and chronic rhinosinusitis.

Patients with traumatic anterior cranial fossa CSF leaks require long-term monitoring for delayed complications including recurrent CSF leakage, infection, and mucocele development. A high index of suspicion for recurrent CSF leakage should be maintained for patients who present with delayed meningitis, and patients should be appropriately counseled on the symptoms of CSF leakage including worsening headaches, constant or intermittent clear nasal drainage, and a persistent sensation of postnasal drip.

Complications and Management

Reported morbidity rates following surgical repair of traumatic CSF leaks, including wound infection, meningitis, abscess formation, seizures, and neurological injury, range from 1.3% to 24.9%, while recurrent CSF leakage rates range from 2% to 20%.[13] An extended period of CSF diversion via lumbar drainage following fistula repair is often utilized to promote closure of the dural defect. The efficacy of lumbar drainage in preventing recurrent CSF leakage remains uncertain, however; patients must be carefully monitored for signs of CSF overdrainage including severe worsening of positional headaches that may indicate development of a subdural hematoma requiring emergent evacuation or cessation of CSF diversion. In the setting of sinus injury and inadequate skull base repair, pneumocephalus may also rapidly develop and be worsened by CSF diversion. Patients with a change in neurological status should have repeat imaging to ensure that the pneumocephalus is not under tension (Figure 11.3).

Mucocele development after a fracture of the frontal sinus is an uncommon but well-recognized complication that may occur after both surgical and nonsurgical management. Mucoceles may present many years after the traumatic injury and are frequently caused by

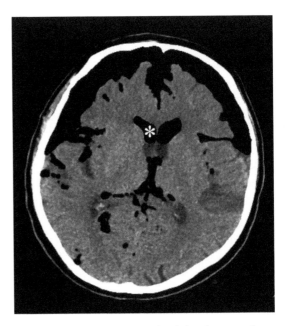

Figure II.3 Axial CT demonstrating bilateral subdural areas of pneumocephalus with frontal lobe compression and intraventricular pneumocephalus (*).

persistent mucous production within the frontal sinus with outflow obstruction. This obstruction may be the sequelae of the initial traumatic injury or result from surgical obliteration of the frontal sinus with inadequate mucosa exenteration.[14] Nondisplaced fractures of the posterior wall of the frontal sinus are not thought to significantly predispose to a higher incidence of mucocele formation, but long-term surveillance is necessary. Endoscopic endonasal surgery for CSF repair may also lead to mucocele formation via inflammation and resultant stenosis of the sinus outflow tract.[15] Both endoscopic and open techniques have shown good efficacy in treating patients presenting with symptomatic mucoceles by restoring sinus outflow or performing complete obliteration of the sinus.

Oral Boards Review: Complications Pearls

- Beware of CSF overdrainage while treating a leak by CSF diversion.
- Tension pneumocephalus may require urgent surgical treatment.
- Patients with endoscopic repair require sinus precautions (head of bed >30 degrees, no nose blowing/sneezing/Valsalva maneuvers, and no nasogastric tube placement without direct visualization).
- Patients may require long-term follow-up for surveillance of possible recurrent leak, infection, or mucocele development.

Evidence and Outcomes

Meningitis is one of the most devastating potential consequences of traumatic CSF leaks. The use of prophylactic antibiotics in patients with CSF leak remains controversial, and multiple retrospective studies have shown no difference in the incidence of meningitis with the use of prophylactic antibiotics. A Cochrane review that included 208 patients from four randomized controlled trials did not support the use of antibiotics to reduce the risk of meningitis.[16] Patients with traumatic CSF leaks that persist for more than 7 days experience a dramatic increase in their incidence of meningitis. Thus, for patients in whom initial conservative measures fail, surgical intervention is recommended to decrease the risk of infection.

Both endoscopic endonasal and open transcranial surgical approaches are effective in resolving traumatic CSF leaks from the anterior cranial fossa, with reported success rates ranging from 90% to 98% using the endoscopic approach and 86% to 97% for open transcranial approaches.[2,7,10]

References

1. Oh JW, et al. Traumatic cerebrospinal fluid leak: Diagnosis and management. *Korean J Neurotrauma.* 2017;13(2):63–67.

2. Banks CA, Palmer JN, Chiu AG, O'Malley BW Jr, Woodworth BA, Kennedy DW. Endoscopic closure of CSF rhinorrhea: 193 cases over 21 years. *Otolaryngol Head Neck Surg.* 2009;140:826–833.

3. Meco C, Oberascher G, Arrer E, et al. Beta-trace protein test: New guidelines for the reliable diagnosis of cerebrospinal fluid fistula. *Otolaryngol Head Neck Surg.* 2003;129:508–517.

4. Zapalac JS, Marple BF, Schwade ND. Skull base cerebrospinal fluid fistulas: A comprehensive diagnostic algorithm. *Otolaryngol Head Neck Surg* 2002;126:669–676.

5. Mostafa BE, Khafaqi A. Combined HRCT and MRI in the detection of CSF rhinorrhea. *Skull Base.* 2004;14:157–162.

6. Lin DT, Lin AC. Surgical treatment of traumatic injuries of the cranial base. *Otolaryngol Clin North Am.* 2013;46(5):749–757.

7. Phang SY, et al. Management of CSF leak in base of skull fractures in adults. *Br J Neurosurg.* 2016;30(6):596–604.

8. Yilmazlar S, Arslan E, Kocaeli H, et al. Cerebrospinal fluid leakage complicating skull base fractures: Analysis of 81 cases. *Neurosurg Rev.* 2006;29:64–71.

9. Eljamel MS, Foy PM. Acute traumatic CSF fistulae: The risk of intracranial infection. *Br J Neurosurg.* 1990;4:381–385.

10. Senior BA, Jafri K, Benninger M. Safety and efficacy of endoscopic repair of CSF leaks and encephaloceles: A survey of the members of the American Rhinologic Society. *Am J Rhinol.* 2001;15:21–25.

11. Kirtane MV, Gautham K, Upadhyaya SR. Endoscopic CSF rhinorrhea closure: Our experience in 267 cases. *Otolaryngol Head Neck Surg.* 2005;132:208–212.

12. Prosser JD, et al. Traumatic cerebrospinal fluid leaks. *Otolaryngol Clin North Am.* 2011;44(4):857–873, vii.

13. Eljamel MS, Foy PM. Post-traumatic CSF fistulae, the case for surgical repair. *Br J Neurosurg.* 1990;4:479–482.

14. Kamoshima Y, Terasaka S, Nakamaru Y, Takagi D, Fukuda S, Houkin K. Giant frontal mucocele occurring 32 years after frontal bone fracture: A case report. *Case Rep Neurol.* 2012;4:34–37.

15. Chen KT, Chen CT, Mardini S, Tsay PK, Chen YR. Frontal sinus fractures: A treatment algorithm and assessment of outcomes based on 78 clinical cases. *Plast Reconstr Surg.* 2006;118:457–468.

16. Ratilal BO, Costa J, Sampaio C. Antibiotic prophylaxis for preventing meningitis in patients with basilar skull fractures. *Cochrane Database Syst Rev.* 2006;(1):CD004884.

Management of Temporal Bone Fractures

Hongzhao Ji and Brandon Isaacson

12

Case Presentation

A 25-year-old man with no past medical history presents with right facial weakness and hearing loss after a motor vehicle collision 4 days ago. He has nondisplaced facial and cervical vertebrae fractures for which he wears a cervical collar. A CT brain scan was performed at an outside hospital showing a right temporal bone fracture. He was hospitalized for 2 days and intubated for less than 24 h during that time. He denies any clear rhinorrhea or otorrhea but reports some bleeding from his ear.

Questions

1. Is the imaging modality used adequate? If not, what other studies should be performed?
2. What are the most important elements of the physical exam for this patient?
3. What other tests should be considered?
4. What is the timing of diagnostic workup?
5. What are the key elements of the history when evaluating traumatic facial paralysis?

Assessment and Planning

An intratemporal facial nerve injury is the suspected mechanism for this patient's facial paralysis. The hearing loss is thought to be secondary to either ossicular chain disruption and/or otic capsule violation. Facial nerve injury can occur along any segment; however, the most common location in the setting of temporal bone trauma is the perigeniculate region.

Hearing loss due to temporal bone trauma can be conductive, sensorineural, or mixed. Ossicular chain disruption and fluid (blood, spinal fluid) in the middle ear space are the most common mechanisms for conductive loss. An otic capsule-sparing fracture with ossicular chain disruption can produce a maximum conductive loss (Figure 12.1). Violation of the otic capsule typically results in profound sensorineural loss (Figure 12.2).

Though not present in this case, CSF leak is also a possible complication associated with temporal bone trauma. Injury to the bone and dura of the middle and posterior fossa within the temporal bone are the typical sites for a traumatic CSF leak. An otic capsule–involving fracture with communication to the subarachnoid space and middle ear is another less common mechanism for traumatic CSF otorrhea. A concurrent perforation

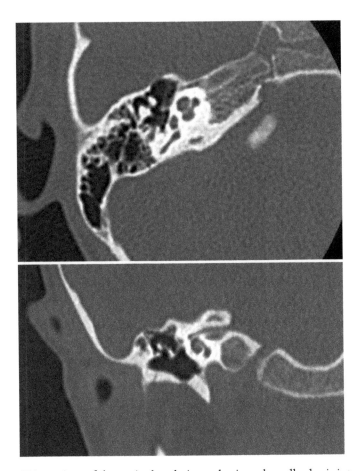

Figure 12.1 Disruption of the ossicular chain at the incudomalleolar joint.

of the tympanic membrane is the typical route for CSF otorrhea, whereas rhinorrhea occurs in the setting of an intact tympanic membrane via the Eustachian tube.

CSF leak, facial nerve injury, hearing loss, great vessel injury, and vestibular dysfunction are all potential complications of temporal bone trauma. Awareness of all of these complications and the overlap between their management is key to comprehensive care for temporal bone fractures.

Oral Boards Review: Diagnostic Pearls

- Physical exam is critical, especially in the acute setting.
  - *Otoscopy.* Ear canal lacerations often heal without intervention; however, circumferential lacerations can potentially cause stenosis of the canal with scarring. Hemotympanum is a common finding, representing blood in the middle ear space. Perforation in the tympanic membrane can also be seen, and CSF leak can be observed at times.
  - *512 Hz tuning fork.* The Weber test involves placing a vibrating tuning fork against a bony prominence in the midline of the head. Sound will be heard on the side with a conductive hearing loss or opposite from the side with a sensorineural hearing loss. A Rinne test compares air conduction

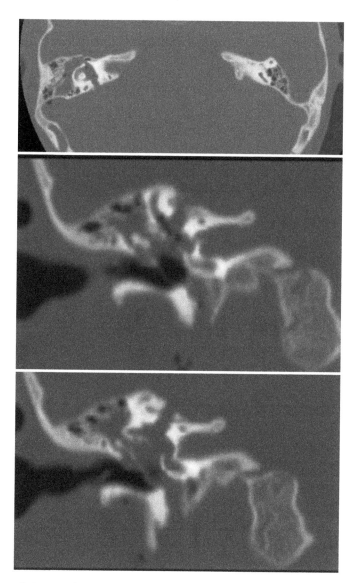

Figure 12.2 Otic capsule disrupting fracture on the right.

by holding a tuning fork next to an ear and then comparing the perceived volume to bone conduction by holding the fork against the mastoid on the same side. Bone conduction louder than air conduction suggests conductive loss.

- *Facial movement.* The House–Brackmann scale is a simple grading system for reporting the level of facial nerve function, with 1 indicating normal function and 6 indicating total paralysis. House–Brackman 1 or 2 is considered adequate recovery in most resources and publications.

- *Oculomotor exam.* Disruption of the otic capsule typically presents with symptoms of dizziness and vertigo and exam findings of nystagmus, imbalance, and a positive head impulse test. A head impulse test is a simple method for assessing semicircular canal function. Lateral gaze paresis or ophthalmoplegia may be present with more extensive skull base injuries secondary to oculomotor or abducens nerve injuries respectively.

- *CSF leak.* This usually involves a persistent or intermittent drainage of clear fluid from the nose or ear. Leaning the patient forward with the head down for 60 sec can often unmask an occult CSF leak.
- An audiogram is an essential diagnostic study for patients with temporal bone fractures. *Audiometry* is often delayed for several weeks after the initial injury to allow for resolution of middle ear fluid unless the patient requires more urgent surgical intervention. Audiometry provides an objective means of categorizing the degree and type of hearing loss. *Tympanometry*, usually done in conjunction with the audiogram, can also suggest presence of fluid in the middle ear space.
- *Immediate versus delayed weakness.* Facial nerve weakness is not always immediate in onset. Documenting facial function as soon after the injury as possible helps guide management but is often delayed secondary to loss of consciousness and/or other injuries taking priority. Those patients who cannot be examined immediately must be considered to have an indeterminate onset of paralysis. Patients with delayed-onset weakness have a more favorable prognosis for recovery.
- *Complete versus incomplete.* Incomplete paralysis recovery is nearly 100%.
- *Imaging.* High-resolution temporal bone CT scan is typically reserved for patients with persistent CSF leaks, hearing loss, or facial paralysis and should also be obtained prior to any surgical intervention. CT imaging is helpful in determining whether the fracture involves the otic capsule.
- *Electromyography and electroneurography.* Electromyography (EMG) is usually performed as a nerve excitability test (NET) in which the stimulation is increased gradually until twitching is seen. This is then compared to the contralateral side. Another test is the maximal stimulation test (MST), in which both sides are stimulated to produce maximum possible contraction and the affected side is subjectively rated for the amount of reduced contraction. Electroneuronography (ENOG) is a bipolar stimulation that quantifies the amount of degeneration in the affected side by comparison to the normal contralateral side. Patients with greater than 90% difference between the involved versus uninvolved ears have a poorer prognosis for facial nerve recovery.
- *Timing of electrodiagnostic testing.* Nerves with neurapraxia maintain stimulability. Nerves with complete disruption will retain distal stimulability for 3–5 days. During this time, the nerve undergoes Wallerian degeneration.

In this case, the exam showed right intact tympanic membrane with hemotympanum, and the Weber test was heard louder on the right. Rinne testing showed bone conduction greater than air conduction bilaterally, consistent with a conductive hearing loss. The onset of the patient's facial paralysis was indeterminate as the patient was found unconscious. Right facial nerve function was rated as a House-Brackmann grade 6.

The patient had EMG and ENOG ordered as well as an audiogram and dedicated temporal bone imaging. Five days after the initial visit, the volitional EMG showed no signal on the right side. The ENOG showed 95% degeneration compared to the contralateral side. A temporal bone CT showed multiple otic capsule–sparing fractures with incudo-malleolar discontinuity and a fracture traversing the perigeniculate facial nerve. An audiogram showed a flat tympanogram on the right and a moderate conductive hearing loss on the right with normal hearing on the left.

The patient denied any clear otorrhea or rhinorrhea in this case, suggesting no active CSF leak. CSF leak is most often seen through a defect in the tegmen tympani or tegmen mastoideum for otic capsule–sparing fractures and more rarely through a fistula from the posterior cranial fossa into the disrupted otic capsule.

β2-transferrin can be used to test collected fluid to confirm the presence of a CSF leak. High-resolution imaging can also be used to localize the site of the leak. When other methods fail, fluorescein dye can be mixed with collected CSF from a lumbar drain and injected back into the patient to localize the site of the leak. A persistent CSF leak increases the risk of developing bacterial meningitis.

Questions

1. What are factors indicating poor prognosis for facial nerve recovery?
2. What are the possible findings on Weber and Rinne tuning fork tests, and what are their significance?

Decision Making

Facial Nerve Injury

Surgical decompression is recommended for complete and immediate-onset facial nerve paralysis with a poor prognosis for recovery based on volitional and evoked EMG. In this case, the patient was treated as having indeterminate onset with complete paralysis and unfavorable electrodiagnostic results.

Hearing Loss

A persistent conductive hearing loss lasting longer than 6–12 months can be addressed with an exploratory tympanotomy with possible ossiculoplasty, continued observation, or with amplification. Surgical middle ear exploration in the period immediately following the injury is not recommended as scar formation around the ossicular chain and resorption of middle ear fluid often results in resolution or improvement in the patient's hearing loss.

Cerebrospinal Fluid Leak

Traumatic CSF leaks often resolve with conservative measures within 1 week after the initial injury. Conservative treatment includes stool softeners, head of bed elevation, and refraining from exertion. Leaks that persist can be treated with a lumbar drain, but there is no clear consensus on how long a patient should be observed prior to a lumbar drain trial. Patients who have a persistent leak despite an adequate trial of lumbar drainage should undergo surgical repair.

Surgical decompression of the facial nerve as well as ossicular chain reconstruction was recommended to this patient given his poor prognosis for recovery. The patient agreed and was taken to the operating room for surgery the following day (10 days after initial trauma). Regardless of the treatment recommended, systemic steroid therapy should be considered in patients with facial nerve weakness or sensorineural hearing loss.

Questions

1. In a patient who could not be examined immediately after injury, should they be treated as delayed or immediate onset?
2. Should surgical exploration be carried out on a patient with incomplete paralysis?
3. Is antibiotic prophylaxis needed for a temporal bone fracture without CSF leak?
4. What is the range of timing for CSF leak after a temporal bone trauma?

Surgical Procedure

Complications of temporal bone trauma must be considered together to synthesize a surgical plan for intervention. Presence or absence of sensorineural hearing loss is one of the main factors that determines the surgical approach.

Surgical decompression of the facial nerve is done under general anesthesia. The surgical approach used for facial nerve decompression is determined by the patient's hearing status and the location of the injury. A translabyrinthine approach provides access to the entire intratemporal facial nerve for patients with a profound sensorineural hearing loss. For patients with intact cochlear function, a combined transmastoid middle fossa approach is the procedure of choice. The distal labyrinthine and perigeniculate facial nerve can be decompressed using a transmastoid supralabyrinthine approach which often requires removal of the incus and malleus head. Ossicular chain reconstruction is necessary to address the conductive hearing loss. In cases of severe middle ear mucosa inflammation, ossicular chain reconstruction can be staged.

The patient is placed in the supine position with the head turned away from the affected side. A facial nerve monitor is placed because it can provide information on the state of the nerve with stimulation, provided surgery is performed within 72 h of the initial injury. The incision should be placed in the postauricular region, with the entire affected side of the head and scalp prepped if a middle cranial fossa approach becomes necessary. The middle cranial fossa approach can also be useful in repairing tegmen defects in patients with persistent CSF leakage.

Facial nerve decompression begins with a mastoidectomy. The antrum is exposed, along with the lateral semicircular canal. The fallopian canal is opened, and, in the process, the mastoid segment of the facial nerve is skeletonized. The incus buttress is taken down, and the tympanic segment can be accessed and skeletonized. A supralabyrinthine approach is then taken to expose the distal labyrinthine segment. Traumatized segments of the facial nerve are exposed; however, the nerve sheath is preserved whenever possible.

Short-term surgical intervention for conductive hearing loss is usually not indicated as the resultant conductive hearing loss will often improve secondary to scar formation.

The surgical approach for persistent CSF leak depends largely on the location of the leak. Anterior skull base leaks should be repaired from a nasal approach with mucoperichondrial flap. Leaks from otic capsule–disrupting fractures can be managed with obliteration of the middle ear and Eustachian tube with closure of the ear canal. Otic capsule–sparing fractures are often addressed via a transmastoid approach, but a middle cranial fossa approach may become necessary to facilitate repair. A conchal or tragal cartilage graft can be used for small skull base defects. A temporalis flap can be used to provide coverage for larger skull base defects.

Oral Boards Review: Management Pearls

- The perigeniculate facial nerve is the most common site of injury in patients with facial paralysis secondary to temporal fractures (80–90%).
- A significant portion of patients have multiple sites of facial nerve injury.
- Surgical decompression should be discussed with patients with immediate onset and complete paralysis who have unfavorable EMG and ENOG results.
- Systemic steroid therapy is indicated in facial paralysis regardless of surgical intervention
- The tegmen is the most common site of disruption and CSF leak in otic capsule–sparing fractures, while connection from the posterior cranial fossa to the disrupted otic capsule is the source for otic capsule–involving fractures.

Pivot Points

- What approaches should be taken for facial nerve decompression in the case of a patient with profound sensorineural hearing loss? What about in a patient with intact cochlear function?
- What approach should be taken in a case with persistent CSF leak with intact cochlear function? What about with profound sensorineural hearing loss?

Aftercare

The most important aspect of aftercare in patients with facial nerve paralysis is eye care. Inability to close the eye and blink effectively can lead to complications including exposure keratitis and corneal abrasions. Artificial tears and topical eye ointments are the mainstays of eye care. Taping the upper or lower lid can be considered in addition to wearing a moisture chamber. If done incorrectly, eye care measures can exacerbate a corneal abrasion. If taping is performed, tape should be placed as laterally as possible in order to avoid taping directly over the cornea. An ophthalmology consult should be considered in any patient with chemosis, persistent foreign body sensation in the eye, or vision changes. Patients with persistent diplopia should also be referred to ophthalmology.

Vestibular rehabilitation is also an important aspect of postoperative care in patients with altered vestibular function or in those who have undergone a translabyrinthine surgical exposure. Vestibular rehabilitation with an experienced physical therapist should be initiated as soon as possible.

Follow-up for patients after surgery or after observation should include audiometry. An audiogram is obtained typically 1–3 months after surgery to allow for Gelfoam to dissolve and integration of the prosthesis. Patients who have fractures involving the external auditory canal are at risk for acquired cholesteatomas. Imaging should be performed 6–12 months after surgery to assess for this if a staged, second-look procedure is not already planned.

Facial nerve recovery time is variable, taking place anywhere from 1 day to 1 year after decompression. Adequate time (1 year) should be allowed to pass before referral for facial reanimation.

Persistent CSF leak should be monitored. In cases where there is high flow or risk for continued leak, a lumbar drain can be retained for a longer period of time.

Complications and Management

Persistent facial nerve weakness that does not return after surgical decompression or cable grafting can be managed with facial reanimation surgery. The most important consideration is eye protection. This can be accomplished by placement of an upper eyelid weight and/or a tarsal strip and pexy. Eye ointment is often still necessary to maintain moisture.

A persistent CSF leak will require surgical repair if conservative management or lumbar drainage fail to resolve this issue. There is some evidence for antibiotic prophylaxis in the setting of CSF leak, but no consensus protocol of prophylaxis has been established. Meningitis can be a complication of CSF leak, which must be treated with appropriate culture-directed antibiotics if bacterial. The most common bacteria are *H. influenzae* and *S. pneumoniae*.

Cholesteatoma is a potential postoperative complication after any ear surgery or temporal bone trauma. Traumatic implantation of skin epithelium into the middle ear can occur at the time of fracture. Fractures involving the canal can lead to canal cholesteatoma as well. If the patient's surgery is staged, a thorough examination of the middle ear should be performed to look for evidence of cholesteatoma. Postoperative or posttraumatic external canal stenosis can disrupt hearing as well as reduce access for surveillance of the ear.

Oral Boards Review: Complication Pearls

- Vestibular deficits require consistent work with physical therapy. There should always be consideration for a third window in the vestibular system.
- Carotid canal fracture is moderately sensitive and specific for carotid artery injury. Carotid angiography should be obtained in any patient with

neurological symptoms not otherwise explained, lateralizing symptoms, or a displaced fracture involving the carotid canal or cervical bruit.

- Eye protection should be a first priority in persistent facial nerve weakness.
- There should always be suspicion for cholesteatoma, which may take years to present. MRI with diffusion weighted imaging can detect cholesteatomas as small 3 mm.

Evidence and Outcomes

Data comparing intervention and observation are rare, being mostly observational studies or case series. Studies directly comparing observation to surgical intervention are difficult to control. There is good evidence that most facial nerve injuries will recover even in patients with immediate-onset complete paralysis. There are no data supporting or condemning the use of corticosteroids in the setting of facial nerve injury; however, the practice remains common due to the theoretical mechanism behind progressive facial weakness. There is abundant observational evidence for the most common locations of facial nerve injury being the perigeniculate and mastoid segment. Adequate studies comparing surgical to nonsurgical intervention are still lacking, and recommendations can be controversial.

Evidence for CSF leak, like much of temporal bone fracture management, is comprised mostly of observational data and lacks well-controlled studies. β2-transferrin has been studied and shown to be a good test when assessing for CSF leak. The vast majority of traumatic CSF leaks will close spontaneously. While many individual studies showed little evidence for prophylactic antibiotics in the setting of a CSF leak, a meta-analysis showed benefit.

Further Reading

Brodie HA. Prophylactic antibiotics for posttraumatic cerebrospinal fluid fistulae. A meta-analysis. *Arch Otolaryngol Head Neck Surg.* 1997;123(7):749–752.

Brodie HA, Thompson TC. Management of complications from 820 temporal bone fractures. *Am J Otology.* 1997;18(2):188–197.

Dahiya R, Keller JD, Litofsky NS, Bankey PE, Bonassar LJ, Megerian CA. Temporal bone fractures: Otic capsule sparing versus otic capsule violating clinical and radiographic considerations. *J Trauma.* 1999;47(6):1079–1083.

Grant JR, Arganbright J, Friedland DR. Outcomes for conservative management of traumatic conductive hearing loss. *Otology neurotology.* 2008;29(3):344–349.

Nash JJ, Friedland DR, Boorsma KJ, Rhee JS. Management and outcomes of facial paralysis from intratemporal blunt trauma: A systematic review. *Laryngoscope.* 2010;120(7):1397–1404.

Orbital Trauma

Aaron R. Plitt, Benjamin Kafka, Tarek Y. El Ahmadieh,
and Christopher J. Madden

13

Case Presentation

A 10-year-old girl presented to the trauma hall after being involved in a motor vehicle collision. The patient was a back-seat passenger and required extrication from the vehicle by bystanders. On arrival of the EMS team, the patient was combative and required sedation followed by intubation. On initial examination, it was noted that the patient had significant left periorbital ecchymosis and edema as well as a palpable depression to the left frontal skull superior to the left eye. Her globe was intact on the left. There was also dried blood over the face and in the bilateral nares and a laceration to the lower lip. The pupils were small but reactive. There were no other abnormalities on physical exam, but the exam was limited due to recent sedation and intubation.

> **Questions**
>
> 1. What is the most appropriate next step?
> 2. What are the most appropriate imaging modalities?
> 3. What are the most appropriate anatomical areas to image and why?
> 4. What must be ruled out when evaluating orbital trauma?

Assessment and Planning

Due to the high-impact mechanism of injury, the palpable fracture line in the left frontal skull, and the limited history, a CT of the head and face was obtained. This revealed a complex comminuted fracture of the left superior and lateral orbital rims and zygomatic arch, as well as the greater wing of the sphenoid bone with possible impingement on extraconal contents as well as a left frontal hematoma and scattered subarachnoid hemorrhage (Figure 13.1). Neurosurgery, ENT, oral-maxillofacial surgery, and ophthalmology were consulted to evaluate the patient's multiple injuries.

> **Questions**
>
> 1. What is the most appropriate next step in management?
> 2. When would surgery be appropriate?
> 3. What are concerning signs requiring emergent intervention?

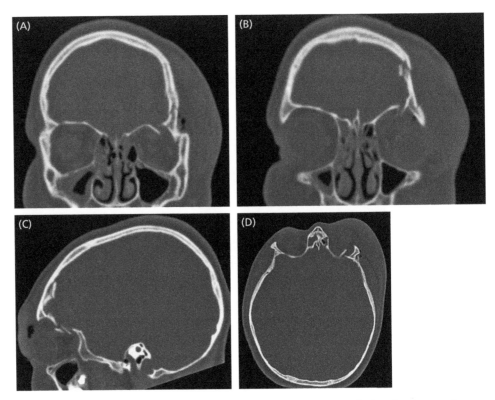

Figure 13.1 (A,B) Coronal, (C) Sagittal and (D) Axial views of a head computed tomography scan demonstrating the left orbital roof fracture with a bony spur projecting into the left orbit.

Oral Boards Review: Diagnostic Pearls

- CT of the head and face should be obtained when there is a high-impact injury to the head and neck.
- Ecchymosis and edema around the eye should be highly suspicious for an orbital fracture.

Decision Making

Orbital and ocular injuries occur at a frequency of 10–17% in the setting of trauma.[1–3] On initial assessment in a trauma setting, the providers should initially ensure the safety of the airway and hemodynamic stability. During the secondary survey, external signs of trauma (e.g., ecchymoses, edema, lacerations) to the head and face should create a high level of suspicion for an orbital injury, such as this patient's palpable fracture line in the frontal bone and the periorbital edema and ecchymosis.

As in this patient, ocular examination may be difficult in a patient with a depressed level of consciousness. In this emergent setting, the integrity of the globe is the most important thing to assess because a ruptured globe is a surgical emergency. Signs of globe rupture include subconjunctival hemorrhage, pupillary shape abnormality, and flattening of the anterior chamber.[1,2] Globe disruption is a surgical emergency, and the patient should be taken to the operating room as soon as possible. The oculocardiac reflex may be elicited in an orbital fracture due to entrapment of the extraocular muscles, which can result in bradycardia, vomiting, syncope, and even asystole.[4] This is also an indication for emergent surgery. These clinical situations were ruled out in this case; therefore, a more thorough physical exam can proceed without need for emergent surgical intervention. An ophthalmology consult is prudent to aid in the examination as well.

The awake patient may complain of diplopia, pain, and nausea, but this was limited in this patient and is commonly limited in the setting of trauma. The physical exam for assessment of orbital injuries should evaluate for symmetry, depth of the globe, position of the globe within the orbit, the ability to open and close the lid, and pupillary assessment. Signs of orbital injury include enophthalmos, hypoglobus, telecanthus, proptosis, periorbital ecchymosis, hypesthesia of the infraorbital nerve distribution, and subcutaneous emphysema.[1–3] The signs present in this case were subcutaneous emphysema and periorbital ecchymosis.

A bedside ophthalmoscope may be utilized for further assessment. It can be used to assess pupillary reactivity, as well as to view the fundus for optic pallor suggestive of optic nerve injury, vascular disruption, or retinal injury (e.g., detachment, tear).

With signs indicating an orbital fracture, the next step in evaluation is obtaining imaging. The preferred modality to assess for orbital fractures is CT. The mnemonic BALPINE has been employed to assist in radiographic assessment for orbital fracture.[3] It stands for bones, anterior chamber, lens, posterior to the globe, intraconal orbit, neurovascular structures, and extraocular muscles/extraconal orbit. An additional metric is the orbital volume because a fracture can expand the space.[1]

After establishing the existence of a fracture, ocular motility should be assessed. Fracture through any wall in the orbit can lead to herniation of the recti muscles and entrapment, which would be an indication for earlier surgical intervention. The most common complaint is diplopia.[1,5] The patient will be unable to move the globe in the direction of action of the entrapped muscle and may report pain with movement. In the unconscious patient, forced duction testing may be used. Along with the motility examination, visual acuity should be assessed.[1,5] Patients with radiographic and/or clinical evidence of entrapment should undergo surgical intervention within 48 h to prevent permanent diplopia.[5]

In the absence of entrapment or globe rupture, the subject of repair of orbital fractures is debated. The standard management is with observation until approximately 5–14 days after the injury to allow for decreased periorbital edema.[1] Indications for surgery are enophthalmos (>2 mm), persistent ocular motility dysfunction, and persistent diplopia in primary gaze or reading position, CT findings of more than 50% of floor involvement, progressive V2 hypesthesia, and abnormal forced duction testing.[1,6,7] Delaying surgery may also decrease the risk of possible compartment syndrome.[1]

In this case presentation, there was no evidence of globe disruption or entrapment; therefore, the decision was made to pursue standard care with delayed operative fixation to allow at least partial resolution of the extensive facial edema.

The patient was extubated 2 days after admission and remained stable. Eight days after admission, the patient was taken to the operating room for left frontotemporal craniotomy for elevation of depressed skull fracture and repair of frontal orbital deformity.

Questions

1. What are the signs and symptoms of orbital injury?
2. What is the time frame for surgery in orbital fractures?
3. What are the radiographic features to assess when evaluating an orbital injury?

Surgical Procedure

The goal of the surgical intervention is to restore the contours of the bony orbit and restore the orbital volume to normal size, which allows for a more cosmetic and functional result. It can be performed in conjunction with ophthalmology, oral-maxillofacial surgery, ENT, and neurosurgery depending on the location of the fracture. During the surgery there should be adequate exposure of the fracture fragments to allow for proper reconstruction.

In this example, the patient had fractures in the superior and lateral orbital walls extending into the sphenoid wing, as well as a frontal epidural hematoma. Given the complexity of the fracture and an intracranial hematoma, neurosurgery was the appropriate service to perform the surgical intervention.

The patient was positioned supine with the neck flexed slight. A bicoronal incision was performed with preservation of the periosteum of the calvarium to allow for repair of a cerebrospinal fluid (CSF) leak. This allowed for exposure of the superior, medial, and lateral orbital rims as well as the anterior cranial fossa and the anterior portion of the middle cranial fossa. Focal frontal and temporal craniotomies were performed to access the fracture segments and evacuate a frontal epidural hematoma.

Next, depressed fragments of bone were elevated. The dura was inspected for defects. If there is a dural defect along the anterior cranial fossa floor, then a pericranial graft may be laid between the dura and the bone. If the pericranium is not available, then a synthetic dural on-lay graft made of collagen made be used. The graft will eventually be incorporated into the dura and significantly decrease the risk of CSF leak.

After the dura was inspected, the fracture segments were plated together with titanium plates and screws. At this point in the operation, any full thickness lacerations should be debrided and repaired in a cosmetic fashion.

The fractures were thoroughly irrigated to remove debris. The incision was then closed in a standard multilayer fashion.

There is no evidence to support the use of preoperative antibiotics in orbital fractures. It is recommended, though, to give antibiotics with coverage of skin flora prior to incision in the operating room, and these should be redosed as needed (Figure 13.2).[8]

Oral Boards Review: Management Pearls

- Globe rupture or entrapment is an indication for emergent surgical intervention
- In the absence of globe rupture or entrapment, surgery can be delayed for 1–2 weeks to allow for decrease in periorbital edema. If the patient is asymptomatic or there is less than 50% orbital floor involvement, then surgery is not necessary.

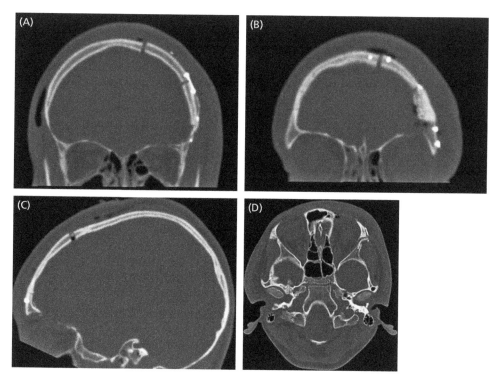

Figure 13.2 (A,B) Coronal, (C) Sagittal and (D) Axial views of a head computed tomography scan demonstrating postoperative fixation of the orbital fracture with good bony alignment.

- The goal of surgery is to restore the normal contour and volume of the orbit.
- There is no role for prophylactic antibiotics in orbital fractures outside of the perioperative period.

Pivot Points

- If a patient presents with signs of globe rupture or entrapment, this is an indication for emergent surgery. Otherwise, surgery can be performed in a delayed fashion.
- CT face is the preferred means of diagnosing an orbital fracture.

Aftercare

Following surgery, the patient was admitted to the hospital for observation. She underwent regular vision checks as well as extraocular motion exams to monitor for the development of complications. This patient received standard perioperative antibiotics for 24 h postoperatively. She did well postoperatively with no diplopia, vision changes, or signs of CSF leak and was discharged to home on the fourth postoperative day after being cleared for safe discharge home by therapists.

Complications and Management

The patient returned to clinic 2 weeks later complaining of intermittent diplopia.

After surgery for orbital fractures, the most common complications are new diplopia, enophthalmos, ectropion, progressive sagging or turning outward of the lower eyelid, and vision loss.[1]

Diplopia following orbital trauma surgery is commonly seen but is rarely permanent and will improve in most cases in a few weeks. The incidence of postoperative diplopia has been reported between 8% and 42%.[1] Given the concern for the hardware, a CT scan of the orbit was obtained while the patient was in clinic. The CT showed a good reconstruction without evidence of entrapment of the extraocular muscles. Therefore, it is likely the postoperative diplopia was caused by direct intraoperative trauma to the extraocular muscles or nerves or progressive fibrosis. It is also more common in older patients, especially when fracture repair is delayed or if there was entrapment or damage to orbital contents.

Postoperative enophthalmos after the repair of orbital fractures is most often caused by inadequate placement of implants and repair of fractures of the orbital cone or by atrophy of the fat within the orbit. The incidence of postoperative enophthalmos is between 7% and 27%.[1] Enophthalmos can be repaired with further surgery by replacing or adding implants but is usually done after the patient has completely healed from the first surgery.

Ectropion postoperatively is most commonly caused by subciliary incisions, and these should be avoided if possible. If ectropion is found postoperatively, the patient must be monitored for dry eyes and aesthetic changes of the eye.

The most concerning postoperative complication following orbital fracture surgery is vision loss. It is usually caused by postoperative intraorbital hemorrhage and has been reported to occur in 0% to 0.4% of cases.[1] If an intraorbital hemorrhage is suspected, then a CT of the face should be obtained emergently to identify the location of the hemorrhage as this will dictate the next step in management. If the hemorrhage occurs in the preseptal space, in relation to the orbital septum, the hemorrhage can be drained or observed depending on the clinical status of the patient. In the setting of new vision loss, drainage should be attempted to restore vision. When the hemorrhage is postseptal and there is new vision loss, increased intraocular pressure, a new afferent pupillary defect, or impaired extraocular movement, a lateral canthotomy and cantholysis should be preformed to protect the orbital tissues from damage resulting from compartment syndrome of the orbit. If pressure in the eye continues to rise despite canthotomy/cantholysis, surgical evacuation of the hemorrhage can be considered.

In the present case, there was no evidence of vision loss or enophthalmos, so she was managed conservatively with observation. Her diplopia slowly resolved over the ensuing 4 weeks.

Oral Boards Review: Complication Pearls

- Diplopia is the most common symptom after orbital fracture repair and is rarely permanent. It should be worked up with a facial CT to evaluate the placement of the hardware and the reconstruction.
- Postoperative vision loss is likely secondary to intraorbital hemorrhage, for which the patient needs a CT of the face. A lateral canthotomy should be performed if there is concern for increased intraorbital pressure followed by surgical evacuation of the hemorrhage.

Evidence and Outcomes

There are few controlled, prospective trials regarding the management of orbital fractures. Most of the evidence comes from case series.

The evidence supports surgical intervention emergently for symptomatic oculocardiac reflex patients and ruptured globes.[1] In the setting of entrapment, operative intervention within 48 h should be considered and is associated with decreased risk of long-term diplopia.[5] In the absence of indications for emergent intervention, delaying surgical intervention for up to 2 weeks is supported in the literature with a small risk of fibrosis and chronic diplopia.[1] The majority of orbital fractures, though, are managed nonoperatively, with patients commonly reporting transient diplopia. Favorable outcomes are obtained in the vast majority of cases. Given the fact orbital fractures are often associated with head trauma, the outcome is often limited by the patient's additional burden of injury.

References

1. Boyette JR, Pemberton JD, Bonilla-Velez J. Management of orbital fractures: Challenges and solutions. *Clin Ophthalmol (Auckland, NZ)*. 2015;9:2127–2137.
2. Ellis E, 3rd. Orbital trauma. *Oral Maxillofacial Surg Clin N Am*. 2012;24(4):629–648.
3. Betts AM, O'Brien WT, Davies BW, Youssef OH. A systematic approach to CT evaluation of orbital trauma. *Emerg Radiol*.2014;21(5):511–531.
4. Kim BB, Qaqish C, Frangos J, Caccamese JF, Jr. Oculocardiac reflex induced by an orbital floor fracture: Report of a case and review of the literature. *J Oral Maxillofacial Surg*. 2012;70(11):2614–2619.
5. Gart MS, Gosain AK. Evidence-based medicine: Orbital floor fractures. *Plast Reconstruct Surg*. 2014;134(6):1345–1355.
6. Burnstine MA. Clinical recommendations for repair of isolated orbital floor fractures: An evidence-based analysis. *Ophthalmology*. 2002;109(7):1207–1210; discussion, 10–11; quiz, 12–13.
7. Burnstine MA. Clinical recommendations for repair of orbital facial fractures. *Curr Opin Ophthalmol*. 2003;14(5):236–240.
8. Mundinger GS, Borsuk DE, Okhah Z, et al. Antibiotics and facial fractures: Evidence-based recommendations compared with experience-based practice. *Craniomaxillofacial Trauma Reconstruct*. 2015;8(1):64–78.

Blunt Cervical Vascular Injury

Aaron R. Plitt, Benjamin Kafka, and Kim Rickert

14

Case Presentation

A 22-year-old woman presented to the emergency department. She was a restrained driver in a motor vehicle crash at highway speed. On exam, she was found to have a complete spinal cord injury at the level of C5. Cervical spine imaging showed a C5–C6 flexion-distraction injury (Figure 14.1). A CT angiogram was performed of the head and neck and revealed occlusion of bilateral vertebral arteries. The patient had no signs of posterior circulation ischemia. She was taken to the operating room for open reduction and internal fixation of her C5–C6 subluxation.

Questions

1. What are the indications for cervical vascular imaging after a trauma?
2. What is the grading scale for cervical vascular injuries?
3. What are the imaging modalities that can be used for vascular imaging?

Assessment and Planning

Cervical cerebrovascular injuries occur in about 1% of patients with blunt trauma.[1,2] Undiagnosed injuries can carry as much as an 80% risk of morbidity or a 40% risk of mortality.[3] Currently, the Eastern Association for the Surgery of Trauma (EAST) recommends screening for all patients who present with any of the following: neurological abnormality unexplained by their diagnosed injuries, epistaxis from a suspected arterial injury, significant blunt head trauma with a Glasgow Coma Scale (GCS) score of 8 or less, a petrous bone fracture, diffuse axonal injury, a cervical spine fracture particularly involving C1–C3 or through the foramen transversarium, a cervical spine subluxation or rotational injury or a LeFort II or III injury.[4]

The vertebral artery originates from the subclavian artery bilaterally. It travels cranially and enters the transverse foramen most commonly at C6 and travels in the transverse foramina of C1–C6 prior to puncturing the dura and becoming the intracranial portion. Any patient with an injury, blunt or penetrating, along this course should be evaluated for vertebral artery injury. In this case, the patient had a cervical spine subluxation, which places the vertebral artery at risk for injury as it is tethered in the foramen transversarium and thus experiences a large shearing force.

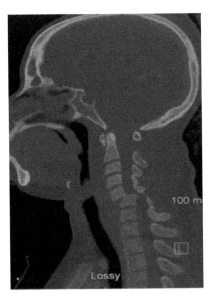

Figure 14.1 Sagittal CT of a C5–C6 flexion/distraction injury.

The gold standard for imaging of cerebrovascular vessels is digital subtraction angiography (DSA).[4] This is an invasive study and not readily available at many centers. Evidence has shown that multislice (eight or greater) multidetector CT angiography (CTA) is as sensitive as DSA for blunt cerebrovascular injury and can be used as a screening tool in patients who meet the selection criteria just listed.[4,5] MR angiography is being used more frequently, especially to evaluate the vessel wall for injury. However, MR angiography is often difficult to obtain for trauma patients and takes longer than a CTA. CTA was chosen for this patient because of the severity of the trauma precluding the need for invasive and time-consuming studies.

Cerebrovascular injuries are graded according to the *Denver scale,* which is a system that was originally proposed by Biffl et al. in 1999.[6]

Grade I: Intimal irregularity with less than 25% narrowing

Grade II: Dissection or intramural hematoma with greater than 25% narrowing

Grade III: Pseudoaneurysm

Grade IV: Occlusion

Grade V: Transection and extravasation

In the present case, vascular imaging showed bilateral grade IV vertebral artery dissections (Figure 14.2).

Questions

1. What is the appropriate treatment for the cervical vascular injuries?

2. What are the indications and risks associated with anticoagulation versus antiplatelet therapy?

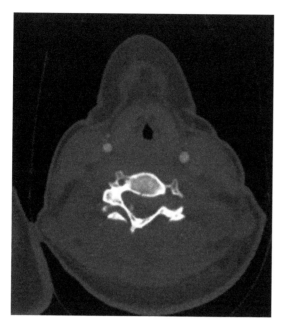

Figure 14.2 CT angiogram at the level of the subluxation shows no filling of either of the vertebral arteries in the transverse foramen.

Oral Boards Review: Diagnostic Pearls

- Many blunt cerebrovascular injuries go undiagnosed due to a lack of vascular imaging and can have serious consequences in the patient's outcome. All trauma patients should be screened by the criteria suggested by EAST, and imaging should be obtained for those patient's who fulfill the criteria.
- Consider a cerebrovascular injury in patients with neurological deficits that are not explained by their already diagnosed injuries.

Decision Making

There are no randomized controlled trials to help guide decision making in the treatment of blunt cervical cerebrovascular injuries. Treatment for a given injury depends on symptoms, site of injury, severity of injury, and other injuries. Vertebral or carotid artery injuries can be treated medically or surgically. The typical treatment is medical with anticoagulation or antiplatelet agents. In the setting of polytrauma, anticoagulation or antiplatelet medications can make management of the trauma patient more complex. In addition, the optimal agents, doses, and duration of treatment are unknown, but treatment with antiplatelet agents has been shown to be at least equivalent to treatment with anticoagulation.[7]

Anticoagulation usually consists initially of a heparin drip, and if a heparin drip is used, EAST recommends the drip be started without a bolus. There is also not enough evidence to recommend a titration goal for the activated partial thromboplastin time. The heparin should eventually be converted to an oral anticoagulant. If warfarin is chosen, the goal INR should be 2–3. This anticoagulation should be continued for 3–6 months.[4] Hemorrhagic complications of heparin in the setting of polytrauma may range from 8% to 16%.[8]

On the other hand, antiplatelet agents are easier to administer compared to a heparin drip. They are usually well tolerated by the trauma patient. In one study, there were no major adverse events attributable to aspirin, and, in two additional studies, there was a lower risk of hemorrhage in patients treated with aspirin compared to anticoagulation.[9–11] Therefore, many large-volume trauma centers have moved to treating cervical vascular injuries with antiplatelet agents.

An additional consideration is the timing of the initiation of the antiplatelet/anticoagulation. In the present case, the patient has an unstable cervical spine requiring operative reduction, fixation, and bony fusion. Anticoagulant use, as stated previously, has a higher rate of hemorrhagic complications. Antiplatelets have a theoretical risk of decreasing fusion rate, but this has not been shown in the literature. Given the fact that this patient is young, though, and should have a robust fusion, the choice was made to initiate aspirin in the perioperative period. It was begun postoperatively because the patient was taken from the trauma hall to the operating room emergently. Zhang et al. performed a meta-analysis revealing no increased risk of intraoperative blood loss in spine surgery with aspirin use.[12] Thus, it would have been safe to start aspirin preoperatively.

Endovascular intervention provides additional treatment options. Again, there are no randomized controlled studies suggesting that endovascular treatment is superior or inferior to best medical management. Stent placement for the treatment of a carotid or vertebral artery dissection is becoming more widely accepted. Stenting allows for re-construction of the internal vessel wall and eventual healing of the dissection. Stenting can also help restore the luminal diameter. This can be beneficial in a patient who is symptomatic secondary to a decrease in flow through a narrow artery. Coiling or stent/coiling of a pseudoaneurysm can possibly decrease the risk of thrombus forming in a pseudoaneurysm and subsequent artery-to-artery emboli. It is important to remember that if a stent is used in endovascular repair, then the patient will need to be placed on dual antiplatelet agents for a period of time postprocedurally. In the case of completely occluded arteries (grade IV), there are reports of occluding the artery with coils prox-imal to the traumatic occlusion to decrease the risk of distal clot migration, but there is no evidence to suggest that this is beneficial.

Given the fact the patient in the presented case was asymptomatic from the vertebral artery occlusions, endovascular treatment was not sought.

Questions

1. Is the patient safe to undergo cervical spine stabilization?
2. When should antiplatelet medications be started?

Surgical Procedure

The trauma patient with cerebrovascular injury often needs cervical spine stabilization, like the patient in this case presentation. Some surgeons worry that manipulation of the neck during surgical fusion may result in dislodging a clot in the artery and cause emboli and a resulting stroke. An analysis of 52 vertebral artery occlusions undergoing cervical fusion done by Foreman et al. suggested that surgery may be protective against stroke and that surgery did not result in increased risk of stroke.[13]

The patient was taken to the operating room within 24 h of the injury. She was placed in a Mayfield head holder and positioned prone on an OSI table. A midline cervical incision was made and the cervical spine was exposed. The subluxation was readily apparent. A C5–C6 laminectomy was performed to evaluate for an epidural hematoma and there was none present. Then the subluxation was partially reduced manually. Lateral mass screws were placed from C2 to C6, and pedicle screws were placed at T1 and T2. The screws were connected with titanium rods bilaterally. The bony surface was then decorticated using a high-powered drill. An artificial bone graft was packed laterally over the lateral masses. The incision was then closed with a subfascial drain in place.

Oral Boards Review: Management Pearls

- Anticoagulation or antiplatelet agents both appear to be reasonable options in the treatment of cervical cerebrovascular injuries.
- There are no studies on correct dosing or length of treatment.
- Serial imaging is warranted because the pathology can be dynamic.

Pivot Points

- Patients presenting with traumatic cervical spine fractures should have a vascular imaging study performed at time of presentation, preferably a CT angiogram of the head and neck.
- The treatment should entail either anticoagulation or antiplatelet therapy.
- Reduction of a fracture-dislocation does not increase the risk of stroke in vertebral artery injury.

Aftercare

The patient should be monitored closely for signs of stroke or hemorrhagic complications postoperatively. The subfascial drain is typically removed within 2–3 days after surgery. The first repeat CTA of the neck is done 1 week after the injury. Blunt vascular injuries can be dynamic, and it is possible for the grade of the injury to change on serial imaging. The optimal length of treatment for antiplatelet agents is unknown. Frequently, with grade I or II injuries, repeat imaging will show resolution of the injury, which may allow the anticoagulation or antiplatelet medications to be stopped.

This patient was monitored in the ICU with spinal cord perfusion protocol. She was started immediately on aspirin 325 mg/d. She had no hemorrhagic complications, and the surgical drain was removed on the third day after surgery. Repeat CTA revealed bilateral grade II vertebral artery dissections at 1 week. She was continued on aspirin for 6 months.

Complications and Management

The most common complications in cerebrovascular injuries are stroke or hemorrhage. Treatment with anticoagulation or antiplatelet agents in a polytrauma patient can result in hemorrhagic complications. It is acceptable to withhold antiplatelet or anticoagulant agents if a complication develops. Warfarin is typically chosen for anticoagulation because it can be reversed readily. Aspirin can be reversed with a platelet transfusion, if indicated.

Oral Boards Review: Complication Pearls

- Stroke or hemorrhage are the two most common complications in patients with cervical cerebrovascular injuries.

Evidence and Outcomes

There are no randomized controlled studies that show diagnosing and treating blunt cervical cerebrovascular injuries is beneficial. There are some case-controlled studies that show that early detection and treatment may help to reduce the risk of stroke and neurological deficit in trauma patients.

References

1. Biffl WL, Ray CE, Jr., Moore EE, et al. Treatment-related outcomes from blunt cerebrovascular injuries: Importance of routine follow-up arteriography. *Ann Surg.* 2002;235(5):699–706; discussion, 7.

2. Miller PR, Fabian TC, Croce MA, et al. Prospective screening for blunt cerebrovascular injuries: Analysis of diagnostic modalities and outcomes. *Ann Surg.* 2002;236(3):386–393; discussion, 93–95.

3. Davis JW, Holbrook TL, Hoyt DB, Mackersie RC, Field TO, Jr., Shackford SR. Blunt carotid artery dissection: Incidence, associated injuries, screening, and treatment. *J Trauma.* 1990;30(12):1514–1517.

4. Bromberg WJ, Collier BC, Diebel LN, et al. Blunt cerebrovascular injury practice management guidelines: The Eastern Association for the Surgery of Trauma. *J Trauma.* 2010;68(2):471–477.

5. Eastman AL, Chason DP, Perez CL, McAnulty AL, Minei JP. Computed tomographic angiography for the diagnosis of blunt cervical vascular injury: Is it ready for primetime? *J Trauma.* 2006;60(5):925–929; discussion, 9.

6. Biffl WL, Moore EE, Offner PJ, Brega KE, Franciose RJ, Burch JM. Blunt carotid arterial injuries: Implications of a new grading scale. *J Trauma.* 1999;47(5):845–853.

7. Cothren CC, Biffl WL, Moore EE, Kashuk JL, Johnson JL. Treatment for blunt cerebrovascular injuries: Equivalence of anticoagulation and antiplatelet agents. *Arch Surg (Chicago, Ill: 1960).* 2009;144(7):685–690.

8. Miller PR, Fabian TC, Bee TK, et al. Blunt cerebrovascular injuries: Diagnosis and treatment. *J Trauma.* 2001;51(2):279–285; discussion, 85–86.

9. Griessenauer CJ, Fleming JB, Richards BF, et al. Timing and mechanism of ischemic stroke due to extracranial blunt traumatic cerebrovascular injury. *J Neurosurg.* 2013;118(2):397–404.

10. Edwards NM, Fabian TC, Claridge JA, Timmons SD, Fischer PE, Croce MA. Antithrombotic therapy and endovascular stents are effective treatment for blunt carotid injuries: Results from long-term followup. *J Am Coll Surg.* 2007;204(5):1007–1013; discussion, 14–15.

11. Cothren CC, Moore EE, Ray CE, Jr., et al. Carotid artery stents for blunt cerebrovascular injury: risks exceed benefits. *Arch Surg (Chicago, Ill: 1960).* 2005;140(5):480–485; discussion, 5–6.

12. Zhang C, Wang G, Liu X, Li Y, Sun J. Safety of continuing aspirin therapy during spinal surgery: A systematic review and meta-analysis. *Medicine.* 2017;96(46):e8603.

13. Foreman PM, Harrigan MR. Blunt traumatic extracranial cerebrovascular injury and ischemic stroke. *Cerebrovasc Dis Extra.* 2017;7(1):72–83.

Blunt Intracranial Cerebrovascular Injury

Benjamin Kafka, Aaron R. Plitt, and Kim Rickert

15

Case Presentation

A 61-year-old male construction worker fell from a 15-foot scaffold, landing on his head. He complained of vision loss in the left eye and diffuse pain throughout his body. On exam, he had a Glasgow Coma Scale (GCS) score of 15 and had no vision or light perception in the left eye. The left eye was also unreactive, with an afferent pupillary defect. The remainder of his neurological exam was normal. His other traumatic injuries consisted of a right calcaneal and fibular fracture and a left forehead laceration. Given the mechanism of injury, a CT scan of the head was completed showing subdural blood located along the frontotemporal convexity, falx, and along the tentorium; scattered small amounts of subarachnoid blood; and multiple skull fractures involving the frontal sinus, ethmoid, crista galli, cribriform plate and medial orbital wall, and dorsum sella; and a left temporal bone fracture (Figure 15.1A,B).

Because of this patient's fractures of the skull base, a CT angiogram (CTA) was also completed to evaluate for cerebrovascular injury during the trauma evaluation. An incidental, small, left posterior communicating artery aneurysm was identified, but no other vascular abnormalities were noted. The patient was admitted to the ICU for observation given the findings of multiple cranial injuries. The patient remained neurologically stable and was cleared to go the operating room for his lower extremity fractures. The patient remained stable and was transferred from the ICU to the ward on hospital day 4. On hospital day 7, he had an acute change in his mental status. On exam he was aphasic and had a right facial droop and right upper extremity weakness.

The patient was transferred to the ICU, labs were drawn, and he was taken for a stat head CT. His sodium levels came back at 120 mmol/L, and the CT showed a left temporal lobe hemorrhage (Figure 15.2). The patient was on prophylactic Lovenox, and this was reversed with protamine. A central line was placed for administration of hypertonic saline. After the patient was stabilized, a CTA of the head was completed due to the location and appearance of the hemorrhage.

Questions

1. What are the criteria for obtaining vascular imaging in trauma?
2. What is the most appropriate initial imaging?
3. Where are the most common intracranial vascular traumatic injuries?

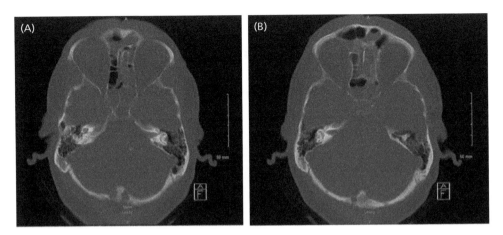

Figure 15.1 CT demonstrating fractures of the ethmoid bone and the left temporal bone (A) as well as the frontal sinus and cribriform plate (B).

Assessment and Planning

Intracranial vascular injury is more common with penetrating injuries than with blunt trauma. As in this patient, cerebrovascular injuries in blunt trauma typically occur where the vessels are located near fracture sites or where they are transitioning from a fixed position (e.g., the carotid canal in the temporal bone) to a more mobile position (e.g., intracranially). Injury can also be seen in vessels along the dural edges (anterior cerebral artery injury in subfalcine herniation), possibly related to traumatic movement of the artery against a relatively fixed dura.[1] The exact incidences of intracranial blunt vascular injuries are not well defined. Traumatic pseudoaneurysms are rare and account for less than 1% of all intracranial aneurysms.[1] They can be associated with morbidity and mortality rates as high as 50%.[1] Therefore, in patients with significant skull base fractures, as in this situation, it is prudent to obtain vascular imaging to evaluate for vascular dissection or pseudoaneurysm. This will allow for early identification of a vascular injury and provide the potential for early intervention.

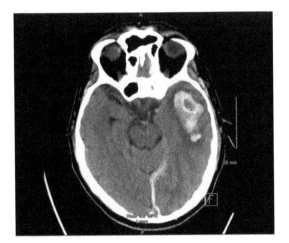

Figure 15.2 CT demonstrating a large left temporal lobe hemorrhage. There is no significant subarachnoid hemorrhage in the basal cisterns.

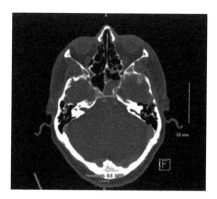

Figure 15.3 CT angiogram shows the pseudoaneurysm of the left middle meningeal artery at the site of the temporal bone fracture.

CTA, MR angiography (MRA), and digital subtraction catheter angiography (DSA) are all studies to evaluate cerebral vasculature. DSA is the gold standard study, but it is an invasive study and not always available to the trauma patient. CTA is relatively quick and can be done at the initial trauma evaluation. It does require intravenous contrast, and, in patients with an allergy to intravenous contrast or poor renal function, MRA might be a better option. The MRA usually takes longer, and a trauma patient might not be able to lie flat for as long as the test takes.

In the present case, the initial CTA showed a left posterior communicating artery aneurysm, and this was thought to be an incidental finding as it was small, berry-shaped, and not in a typical location for a traumatic aneurysm. The second CTA was obtained secondary to the temporal lobe hemorrhage, which identified the delayed development of a left middle meningeal artery pseudoaneurysm of 12 mm (Figure 15.3).

Questions

1. What is the appropriate management of the pseudoaneurysm?
2. Is follow-up vascular imaging necessary in all skull base trauma cases?

Oral Boards Review: Diagnostic Pearls

- Blunt head trauma leading to skull base fractures is associated with a high rate of cerebrovascular injury. All trauma patients with skull base fractures should undergo cerebrovascular imaging with CTA, MRA, or DSA.
- The most common locations of vascular injury are at transition points from fixed to mobile segments or at areas of compression from a fixed structure.

Decision Making

Intracranial vascular injury can happen with different underlying pathologies including dissection of a vessel (usually a larger vessel), formation of a true aneurysm with partial vessel injury leading to a bulge in the weakened vessel wall, or formation of a pseudoaneurysm in which there is a severely weakened wall or vessel rupture contained by a clot and fibrous reaction, and that area is in continuity with the blood flow in the uninjured vessel.

In the case of a dissection, the risks include emboli or formation of a pseudoaneurysm that will lead to rupture. Normally a dissection is treated with antiplatelet or anticoagulation medications to reduce the risk of embolic stroke. Repeat imaging is recommended to assess for change in the vessel.

If there is a traumatic aneurysm or pseudoaneurysm that has ruptured, treatment is indicated. Depending on multiple factors like the condition of the patient and aneurysm location and size, endovascular or surgical treatment options are considered. If the vessel cannot be reconstructed with endovascular or surgical means, then definitive treatment may involve vessel sacrifice. If the pseudoaneurysm is small and has not ruptured, it may be reasonable to treat with antiplatelet or anticoagulant medication and reimage in a short time period to assess for growth or change in the lesion. This is possible, of course, only if there are no systemic contraindications to antiplatelet or anticoagulant therapy. This treatment would seek to minimize any embolic complications associated with the pseudoaneurysm. Growth in the lesion at follow-up imaging generally warrants moving to more aggressive (surgical or endovascular) treatment options.

The natural history of traumatic pseudoaneurysms is not favorable. In 1975, Fleischer et al. reported a 41% mortality rate in patients treated conservatively. This was compared to an 18% mortality rate in patients who were treated surgically.[2] The average time for a pseudoaneurysm to rupture posttrauma was 2–3 weeks.[2] Aggressive treatment is therefore warranted if possible, especially for larger lesions or ones that have hemorrhaged, and the goal of treatment is to exclude the pseudoaneurysm from circulation. Options for treatment of traumatic pseudoaneurysm include craniotomy for clipping, resection or trapping of the aneurysm (with possibility of bypass related to vessel size and location), or endovascular treatment.

Endovascular techniques such as coiling, stent/coiling, vessel sacrifice, or flow diversion have all been successful.[1,3] The choice of treatment depends on both patient and aneurysm factors. In patients who are sicker and not able to tolerate extended anesthesia or with aneurysms that are not easily accessed surgically, endovascular approaches may be better. If a patient has a large hemorrhage that needs to be evacuated simultaneously with fixing the vascular injury, open surgery may be a better option. Due to the rarity of the condition, there are no clinic trials to guide treatment.

Given the location of this patient's pseudoaneurysm in the external carotid circulation and the temporal lobe hematoma, the decision was made to pursue a craniotomy for vessel sacrifice and hematoma evacuation. Evacuation of a temporal lobe hematoma relieves the local mass effect and may improve the patient's neurological outcome.

Questions

1. What are the treatment options for intracranial vessel injury?
2. What are the factors that would argue for more aggressive treatment of a pseudoaneurysm?

Surgical Procedure

The patient was taken to the operating room for a left pterional craniotomy, evacuation of left temporal lobe hematoma, and treatment of the middle meningeal artery aneurysm.

The patient is positioned supine and the head is placed in pins with the Mayfield head-holder. The head is then rotated to the right. A curvilinear incision is made from the root of the zygoma (1 cm anterior to the tragus) to the midline where the hairline typically ends. The temporalis fascia is incised and a single myocutaneous flap is raised anteriorly. Three burr holes are typically made with a perforator drill bit. One at the keyhole, one on the middle fossa floor, and one posteriorly. The burr holes are connected using a craniotome. The bone flap is elevated. At this point, the middle meningeal artery (MMA) will be encountered. Epidural dissection allows for identification of the vessel as it exits foramen spinosum. It can then be ligated with vascular clips.

Then the dura is opened in a c-shape. The hematoma is evacuated with suction and irrigation. Then the dura may be closed, the bone replaced, and the scalp reapproximated.

Oral Boards Review: Management Pearls

- Treatment strategies for cerebrovascular injury include medical, endovascular, or open surgical.
- Medical management of blunt cerebrovascular injury includes antiplatelet and anticoagulation agents. There are no data to suggest that one is better than the other at preventing embolic complications.
- Medical treatment is generally considered for those lesions that are small, not associated with hemorrhage, and/or in locations that do not provide a ready surgical or endovascular option.
- Close follow-up imaging should be obtained to evaluate for progression if medical treatment is pursued.

Pivot Points

- Patients presenting with skull base fractures should undergo an intracranial vascular imaging procedure (CTA, MRA, DSA).
- Delayed neurological decline in a patient with a traumatic brain injury should raise concern for a cerebrovascular injury.
- Treatment for cerebrovascular injury includes endovascular, open surgical, and antiplatelet/anticoagulation therapy depending on factors related to the injury and patient. Incidental injuries may be managed conservatively with close follow-up. Symptomatic injuries will need more aggressive management.

Aftercare

After treatment, the patient was watched in the ICU for 24 h. The patient's right upper extremity strength was near baseline, but his aphasia persisted. A cerebrovascular DSA was completed on postoperative day 1, showing no residual aneurysm. The patient started to work with speech therapy on the first day after surgery. He was eventually discharged on postoperative day 19 to a rehabilitation facility with his only deficit being slow and labored speech. At 2 months follow-up the patient had been discharged from rehab and had full strength throughout and had only a very minor receptive aphasia. Four to six weeks after treatment, the aneurysm was evaluated with a repeat CTA for possible recurrence, which was not found.

In intracranial vessel injury, the patient may be started on aspirin, which may decrease the risk of emboli. This was not done in this situation since the vessel was part of the external carotid circulation.

Complications and Management

A major complication of skull base fractures is the development of a vascular dissection or pseudoaneurysm. A CTA should be considered at the initial presentation of a trauma patient with skull base fractures. Rarely, a vascular injury is initially occult and may develop in a delayed fashion. When a patient with a traumatic head injury has a change in neurological exam after initially improving, there should to be a high suspicion for intracranial hemorrhage and development of a delayed pseudoaneurysm.

Oral Boards Review: Complication Pearls

- Delayed pseudoaneurysm formation should be considered when a patient with blunt head trauma develops a delayed neurological decline.
- Surgical or endovascular repair of a pseudoaneurysm may require vessel sacrifice.

Evidence and Outcomes

There are no randomized controlled studies evaluating the natural history, treatment, or outcomes of patients with traumatic intracranial vessel injuries or traumatic pseudoaneurysms. There is also no strong evidence to support that either delayed angiography or aspirin use are of any benefit or that they may change outcomes in patients with traumatic pseudoaneurysms.[4]

References

1. Larson PS, Reisner A, Morassutti DJ, Abdulhadi B, Harpring JE. Traumatic intracranial aneurysms. *Neurosurg Focus.* 2000;8(1):e4.

2. Fleischer AS, Patton JM, Tindall GT. Cerebral aneurysms of traumatic origin. *Surgical Neurol.* 1975;4(2):233–239.

3. Cohen JE, Gomori JM, Segal R, et al. Results of endovascular treatment of traumatic intracranial aneurysms. *Neurosurgery.* 2008;63(3):476–485; discussion, 85–86.

4. Carney N, Totten AM, O'Reilly C, et al. Guidelines for the management of severe traumatic brain injury, fourth edition. *Neurosurgery.* 2017;80(1):6–15.

Seizures in the Setting of Trauma

Sara Hefton

16

Case Presentation

In the morning, a 71-year-old alcoholic man was found at the bottom of the stairs by his wife. She did not hear him fall but spoke with him at 10 PM the evening prior. When EMS arrived, he did not open his eyes to voice or pain, had no verbal output, and was withdrawing on the left but extensor posturing on the right (Glasgow Coma Score [GCS] 6). In addition, he was noted to have asymmetric pupils, with a left pupil 6 mm and nonreactive and a right pupil 3 mm and reactive. He was intubated and transported to the hospital.

Questions

1. What is the difference between early posttraumatic seizures (PTS) and late PTS?
2. What are this patient's risk factors for early PTS?
3. What are this patient's risk factors for late PTS?

Assessment and Planning

Emergency department visits in the United States for TBI accounted for 2.5 million visits in 2013, with 282,000 hospital admissions. Seizures are a major complication of TBI and occur in 5–12% of patients, with increasing likelihood with worsened TBI severity. PTS can complicate the acute hospitalization by compounding secondary brain injury after TBI by increasing cerebral metabolic demand, worsening hypoxia, increasing intracranial pressure (ICP), and causing ongoing neuronal injury. Seizures that occur within the first 7 days of an injury are considered "early" PTS. These include seizures that occur on impact or at the time of injury, which are also called *immediate seizures*. In severe TBI, up to 25% of early seizures are subclinical and only detected on EEG, with up to 10% of patients developing status epilepticus. "Late" PTS occur more than 7 days after the initial injury. PTS may be generalized, focal, or focal with secondary generalization, though seizures occurring in the first 24 h are more likely to be generalized, and seizures in ICU patients are more likely to be nonconvulsive and focal with secondary generalization. Recurrent late PTS are considered posttraumatic epilepsy (PTE). TBI is the etiology of epilepsy in approximately 5% of epilepsy patients. While all patients who suffer TBI are at risk of developing seizures, seizures are more likely to happen in certain patient populations and conditions. Early

PTS are more likely in patients aged 65 or less, with immediate seizures, chronic alcoholism, initial GCS score of 10 or lower, posttraumatic amnesia lasting more than 30 min, penetrating head injuries, intracranial bleeds (subdural, epidural, and intracerebral hematomas and/or cerebral contusions), and/or linear or depressed skull fractures. In addition, there is an increased risk for early PTS in children, most pronounced under age 7. People older than 65 years with severe TBI, amnestic periods lasting longer than 24 h, intracranial bleeds, multiple cortical or subcortical contusions, early PTS, and surgical instrumentation are more likely to develop late PTS. Late PTS often recur, with up to 86% of patients developing PTE within 2 years, though in some patients with severe TBI the risk of developing PTS is increased compared to the population for more than 20 years after the initial injury. The incidence of PTE is even greater in military personnel than in the civilian population.

In the present case, emergent CT scan demonstrated a large left subdural hematoma with midline shift. He was loaded with fosphenytoin for seizure prophylaxis. After surgical decompression, he was extubated, with only mild right-sided weakness and word-finding difficulties after emergence from anesthesia. On post-injury day 2 he had a seizure, described as initial right face jerking which spread to his to right arm before evolving into a generalized tonic-clonic seizure. His phenytoin level was low; he was given an additional load and his standing dose was increased.

Oral Boards Review: Diagnostic Pearls

- Recognizing risk factors for early and late post-traumatic seizures is essential.
  - *Early PTS.* These are more likely to occur in patients younger than age 65, with an increased risk in children, especially under age 7. They are more likely to occur when patients have immediate seizures, chronic alcoholism, an initial GCS score of 10 or less, posttraumatic amnesia lasting more than 30 min, penetrating head injuries, intracranial bleeds (subdural, epidural, and intracerebral hematomas and/or cerebral contusions), and/or linear or depressed skull fractures.
  - *Late PTS.* These are more likely to occur in patients older than 65 years with severe TBI (GCS ≤8), who have early PTS, amnestic periods lasting greater than 24 h, intracranial bleeds, multiple cortical or subcortical contusions, and/or surgical instrumentation.
- Seizures may present differently based on the time they occur and the illness of patients, though they may be generalized, focal, or focal with secondary generalization.
  - Seizures occurring in the first 24 h are more likely to generalized.
  - Patients in the intensive care unit are more likely to have nonconvulsive seizures or focal seizures with secondary generalization.
- Neuroimaging including CT or MRI should be conducted to determine potential seizure foci.
- EEG may indicate cortical irritability but will not change the management of patients with mild TBI. Continuous EEG in comatose or altered patients may diagnose subclinical seizures or status epilepticus.

Questions

1. What is the most appropriate medication to give to prevent early post-traumatic seizures?
2. Which patients should receive antiepileptic drug (AED) seizure prophylaxis?
3. How long should patients be given AED seizure prophylaxis?

Decision Making

Patients with TBI should have imaging with CT or MRI. Neuroimaging can be used to understand potential foci of seizure; MRI can detect more subtle hemosiderin deposition which may become epileptogenic foci. While epileptiform abnormalities on routine EEG may indicate a propensity for seizure foci, EEG does not change management in noncomatose patients with TBI. However, patients with moderate to severe TBI may benefit from EEG to exclude status epilepticus as an etiology of coma; up to 10% patients with TBI develop status epilepticus, and up to 25% of patients have subclinical seizures. In these patients, continuous EEG may be used to diagnose and monitor the efficacy of ongoing treatment. If patients have atypical seizure semiology, video or ambulatory EEG may also be useful to confirm epileptic correlates with observed events; psychogenic nonepileptic seizures have been reported in survivors of TBI. The 2017 Brain Trauma Foundation Guidelines for the Management of Severe TBI recommend use of phenytoin as AED seizure prophylaxis for 1 week; this recommendation is often extrapolated to include patients with less severe TBI and risk factors for early PTS. Fosphenytoin is often substituted for phenytoin. The guideline recommendation is based on a randomized controlled trial (RCT) that compared placebo to phenytoin with a loading IV dose of 20 mg/kg and ongoing maintenance dosing to obtain a target serum therapeutic goal of $10–20\ \mu g/mL$; levels were checked 1–3 times weekly to maintain therapeutic range. The study demonstrated decreased early PTS but no effect on late PTS. A subgroup analysis demonstrated worsened neurocognitive performance in severe TBI patients exposed to phenytoin 1 month after injury, though this difference did not persist 1 year after injury. Other concerns with using phenytoin include multiple conditions that may cause variable serum drug levels requiring frequent testing, a narrow therapeutic window, drug interactions, and severe side effects including hypotension and Stevens-Johnson syndrome. Because of these concerns, the efficacy and tolerability of alternate AEDs have been evaluated. A meta-analysis of six cohort studies and one low-quality RCT demonstrated similar rates of early PTS with use of phenytoin or levetiracetam. Protocols for the levetiracetam use varied from 20 mg/kg loading dose, a 1,000 mg loading dose, or no loading dose, with maintenance of either 500 mg twice daily or 1,000 mg twice daily. While this evidence is not strong enough to prompt guideline changes, levetiracetam is sometimes used for seizure prophylaxis after TBI. Studies evaluating phenytoin, valproic acid, levetiracetam, carbamazepine, and phenobarbital have been unsuccessful in preventing development of late PTS.

Our patient's mental status did not return to his baseline after his seizure despite optimization of phenytoin. Continuous EEG was started and demonstrated continuous left frontal epileptiform discharges with intermittent evolution into focal seizures and secondary generalization, consistent with status epilepticus.

Surgical Procedure

Timing of surgery or neurosurgical procedures should not affect timing of administration of AED prophylaxis, which should be given as soon as possible in appropriate patients, as discussed in the "Decision Making" section. Anesthesia and surgery are not contraindicated in the setting of seizures without status epilepticus. Status epilepticus should be controlled before nonemergent surgery to allow optimal medication titration with continuous EEG monitoring. Emergency surgery should not be postponed even in the setting of status epilepticus; appropriate anesthesia induces burst suppression and minimizes ongoing neuronal damage. Surgical evacuation of a seizure focus in the setting of trauma is only necessary in the setting of status epilepticus refractory to medical management, as described in the "Complications and Management" section.

Oral Boards Review: Management Pearls

- Prompt initiation of prophylactic AED is indicated in all patients with severe TBI for at least 1 week and should be considered in patients with risk factors and mild or moderate TBI.
- Guidelines recommend phenytoin/fosphenytoin as AED prophylaxis; however, there are weak data to support levetiracetam as an alternate agent.
- Posttraumatic status epilepticus should be treated with initial benzodiazepine, optimization or load of nonsedating AED, and escalation to continuous infusion of second-line agents in intubated patients when necessary.

Pivot Points

- A TBI patient with prolonged coma or altered mental status after resuscitation should be evaluated for subclinical seizures with EEG.
- Patients with late PTS should be maintained on AED for several weeks to months after injury and are at increased risk of developing PTE.
- Status epilepticus not responsive to aggressive medical management may indicate the need for additional surgical evacuation if seizure onset is lesional.

Aftercare

Postoperative TBI patients who do not return to preoperative baseline should be evaluated for subclinical seizures with continuous EEG. Perioperative patients who may not be awake enough to take oral formulations of AEDs should be given IV formulations if possible to minimize missed or late doses, which may increase risk of seizures. If patients are on AEDs without IV formulation and are not awake enough to take medications orally, temporary enteral access should be obtained for administration of AEDs.

Complications and Management

If patients develop seizures despite AED prophylaxis, it is reasonable to ensure therapeutic drug levels and/or to maximize dosing of monotherapy. AEDs should be continued for several months after a clinical seizure. If patients continue to seize despite optimization of monotherapy, additional AEDs with intravenous formulations (valproic acid, fosphenytoin, levetiracetam, phenobarbital) may be helpful to rapidly achieve therapeutic drug levels. In the setting of prolonged seizure lasting more than 5 min, 4 mg doses of lorazepam should be administered to maximum dose of 0.1 mg/kg. If seizures persist, consistent with status epilepticus, continuous infusion of second-line medications like midazolam or propofol may be necessary to achieve seizure suppression; these medications should only be used in intubated patients. If status epilepticus is refractory despite trials of seizure suppression, further neurosurgical evacuation of an epileptic focus (e.g., epidural or subdural hematoma) may be appropriate. For long-term seizure management, it is reasonable to choose AEDs that are tailored to patients to limit drug interactions and side effects based on comorbid conditions and mechanism of drug clearance.

Our patient was given a total of 0.1 mg/kg of lorazepam in 4 mg doses, and he was loaded with levetiracetam; this failed to improve the EEG pattern, and he had to be reintubated for airway protection. A continuous infusion of midazolam was started and titrated until seizure suppression was achieved on EEG. Midazolam was continued to maintain seizure freedom for 24 h, but when it was weaned, seizures returned. Repeat imaging demonstrated recurrence of the frontal aspect of the left subdural hematoma. He underwent repeat clot evacuation with improvement of epileptiform discharges on postoperative EEG. He tolerated the midazolam wean, and his mental status improved. He was extubated and eventually discharged to rehab on dual therapy with levetiracetam and phenytoin.

Oral Boards Review: Complications Pearls

- Patients with late PTS are at high risk for developing PTE.
- Epilepsy medications should be chosen with medical comorbidities in mind. For instance, patients with liver failure may tolerate levetiracetam better than phenytoin or valproic acid.
- Patients with seizures are at risk of increased disability, with potential loss of social, economic, and transportation independence.

Evidence and Outcomes

Development of PTE is a significant source of morbidity in survivors of TBI, with life-changing consequences. Early PTS are a risk factor for late PTS; however, there is still debate over whether early PTS are an independent risk factor for PTE. Late PTS are a risk factor for PTE, with additional seizures occurring in 86% of patients who suffer from an initial late PTS. Subdural hematoma confers additional risk. Because of the high rate of recurrence after an initial late PTS, it is prudent to begin an AED after the first event. The frequency of seizures is predictive of overall severity of PTE; people with more seizures the first year after TBI often continue to have a high seizure burden and are unlikely to have seizure remission. However, remission rates can reach 25–40% in certain populations. PTE is associated with higher hospital and long-term care costs compared to TBI survivors without PTE, and it is a significant cause of morbidity in TBI survivors. Patients with PTE are more likely to have poorer functional and psychosocial outcomes and require dependent modes of transportation. Patients with seizures need to stop driving for their safety and the safety of others; reporting laws and duration of inability to drive vary according to state law. Certain activities, including swimming, cooking, and childcare, may put the patient or others at risk. Some patients may no longer be able to perform previous jobs and require retraining and/or disability assistance. Further study to determine outcomes in patients with PTE is warranted.

Further Reading

Carney N, Totten AM, O'Reilly C, et al. Guidelines for the management of severe traumatic brain injury, fourth edition. *Neurosurgery.* 2017;80(1):6–15. doi:10.1227/NEU.0000000000001432.

Glauser T, Shinnar S, Gloss D, et al. Evidence-based guideline: Treatment of convulsive status epilepticus in children and adults: Report of the Guideline Committee of the American Epilepsy Society. *Epilepsy Curr.* 2016;16(1):48–61. doi:10.5698/1535-7597-16.1.48.

Lowenstein DH. Epilepsy after head injury: An overview. *Epilepsia.* 2009;50 Suppl 2:4–9. doi:10.1111/j.1528-1167.2008.02004.x.

Torbic H, Forni AA, Anger KE, Degrado JR, Greenwood BC. Use of antiepileptics for seizure prophylaxis after traumatic brain injury. *Am J Health Syst Pharm.* 2013;70(9):759–766. doi:10.2146/ajhp120203.

Zimmermann LL, Diaz-Arrastia R, Vespa PM. Seizures and the role of anticonvulsants after traumatic brain injury. *Neurosurg Clin N Am.* 2016;27(4):499–508. doi:10.1016/j.nec.2016.06.001.

Evaluation and Management of Frontal Sinus Fractures

Geoffrey Peitz, Mark A. Miller, Gregory W. J. Hawryluk, and Ramesh Grandhi

17

Case Presentation

An 18-year-old man arrives in the trauma bay via ambulance after launching from a swing and striking his forehead on the ground. He reports severe headache and face pain but denies facial numbness, blurry vision, or diplopia. He denies any preexisting medical conditions, past surgeries, or allergies. On examination the patient has periorbital and frontal ecchymoses and facial edema, and there is sanguineous drainage from the nares. He is alert, slightly confused, with no deficits on cranial nerve examination. Laboratory data are unremarkable. A noncontrast head CT shows a frontal bone fracture extending through the anterior and posterior tables of the frontal sinus with underlying subdural hematoma and trace subarachnoid hemorrhage, as shown in Figure 17.1.

Questions

1. What is the first step in evaluation of this patient?
2. In addition to noncontrast head CT, what additional imaging protocol is appropriate?
3. What additional information is needed regarding the patient's rhinorrhea?

Assessment and Planning

Initial management of patients with head trauma involves performing an Advanced Trauma Life Support (ATLS) primary survey with airway management and resuscitation as needed, and causes of hemodynamic instability such as active extravasation should be addressed. The force required to fracture a frontal sinus ranges from 800 to 2,200 pounds,[1] thus patients often present with concomitant traumatic brain injury (TBI). Appropriate steps, such as intracranial pressure (ICP) monitoring and stepwise management of elevated ICP, should be performed as necessary.

In a hemodynamically and neurologically stable patient, a fine-cut maxillofacial CT with axial, sagittal, and coronal reconstructions is appropriate for further assessment of facial and skull fractures. With regards to the frontal sinus, it is important to evaluate the anterior table, posterior table, and nasofrontal ducts which drain mucosal secretions from the frontal sinus to the middle meatus of the nose. The nasofrontal ducts lie at the medial

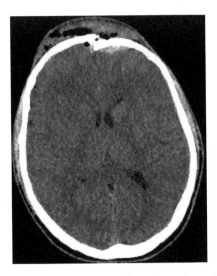

Figure 17.1 Axial head CT without contrast showing a frontal sinus fracture with underlying extra-axial hematoma and traumatic subarachnoid hemorrhage.

floor of the frontal sinuses, and, if obstructed, abscesses or mucoceles can develop within the sinus. Axial and sagittal CT slices are useful for assessing displacement of the anterior and posterior tables, and coronal CT slices are useful for assessing the integrity of the sinus floor and, in some cases, the nasofrontal outflow tract (NFOT). Radiographic criteria associated with NFOT obstruction include sinus floor fractures, medial anterior table (ethmoid air cell wall) fractures, and bone fragments lying in the nasofrontal duct.[2] However, definitive determination of nasofrontal duct obstruction takes place intraoperatively, often by administering fluorescent dye in the frontal sinus and then looking for it in the middle meatus of the nose directly with a nasal speculum or via nasal endoscopy.

Additionally, it is crucial to determine whether the patient has a CSF leak. Blood and mucosal secretions may obscure CSF in gross examination of facial orifice fluid. A systematic review found the "halo" test and CSF glucose and chloride quantification to be unreliable for detecting the presence of CSF in bodily fluid, whereas the presence of β2-transferrin was the most reliable indicator of CSF.[3] Detection of β2-transferrin, which is only present in the CSF and aqueous humor of the globe, by electrophoresis points toward the presence of a CSF leak unless there is a concomitant globe injury.[4] However, it takes 1–3 days for the results of the β2-transferrin test so one must rely on the clinical exam for immediate determination of CSF leak.

In the example patient, maxillofacial CT images showed a right LeFort type II fracture and left LeFort type III fracture as well as a comminuted frontal sinus fracture involving the anterior and posterior table, as shown in Figure 17.2. The fluid at the bilateral nares dried within a few hours after arrival, and there were no further signs of CSF leakage.

Questions

1. What findings on imaging indicate the need for open reduction and internal fixation of a frontal sinus fracture?

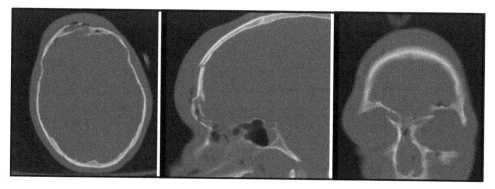

Figure 17.2 From left to right, axial, sagittal, and coronal slices of a noncontrast head CT in bone windows showing displacement of the anterior and posterior tables of the frontal sinus as well as fracture of the sinus floor.

2. In what situations should one cranialize the frontal sinus?
3. Are follow-up appointments or images needed for patients with frontal sinus fractures managed nonoperatively?

Oral Boards Review: Diagnostic Pearls

- Fractures of the floor of the frontal sinus are often associated with nasoorbitoethmoidal fractures, which should be evaluated in their own right to determine appropriate management.
- Up to 25% of frontal sinus fractures are associated with ophthalmologic injury, so a full ophthalmological exam is necessary.
- Identification of a persistent CSF leak is critical because it is the strongest indication for operative management of a frontal sinus fracture.
- In children, the frontal sinus becomes pneumatized between 2 and 8 years of age, and pneumatization continues into adolescence before the frontal sinus is fully developed.

Decision Making

The decision to surgically address a frontal sinus fracture depends on location of the fractures (i.e., anterior table, posterior table or both), displacement of the fracture (where translation of at least the width of the bone qualifies as displaced), and the status of the NFOT (patent or obstructed).[7–9] Anterior table fractures with contour deformities are often reduced and fixated for cosmesis.[10] Significantly displaced posterior table fractures often require surgery to relieve frontal brain compression and repair dural lacerations. An algorithm for management of frontal sinus fractures using these concepts is shown in Figure 17.3. Even in the absence of fracture displacement, NFOT obstruction is an indication for cranialization or, in some cases when only the anterior table is fractured, obliteration of the frontal sinus. If there is anterior table fracture displacement but patency of the NFOT is demonstrated intraoperatively, the sinus may be reconstructed without cranialization or obliteration.

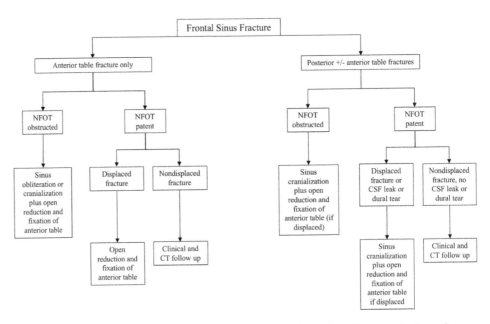

Figure 17.3 Frontal sinus fracture decision-making algorithm. Fractured edges that are translated at least the width of the bone qualify as "displaced." NFOT, nasal frontal outflow tract.

Patients with frontal sinus fractures treated nonoperatively require clinical and radiographic surveillance for the development of CSF leak, mucocele, or infection. The follow-up intervals varies, but clinic visits and maxillofacial CT scans at 3 months, 6 months, then yearly are reasonable.[11]

The patient in our case example had displacement of the anterior and posterior table as well as CT criteria for NFOT obstruction of frontal sinus floor and medial anterior table fractures. The neurosurgeons and oral maxillofacial surgeons planned a joint operation for anterior table open reduction, internal fixation, and cranialization of the frontal sinus.

Questions

1. What type of incision is appropriate for repair of the anterior table only? For cranialization of the frontal sinus?
2. What steps are necessary for cranialization of the frontal sinus?
3. What can be used to seal a cranialized frontal sinus?

Surgical Procedure

Repair of frontal sinus fractures is performed under general anesthesia with a Foley catheter and two routes of IV access. The patient is positioned supine with a horseshoe headrest or occipital cups on a Mayfield bed attachment. Hair may be clipped along the incision or the entire frontal scalp. The scalp and face are prepared with chlorhexidine or Betadine from approximately the coronal suture posteriorly to the superior border of the V2 dermatome anteriorly. Tarsorrhaphy may be performed to protect the corneas

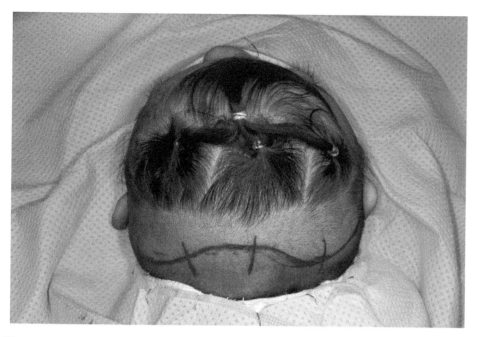

Figure 17.4 Intraoperative photograph of the draping and marked coronal incision for a frontal sinus fracture operation.

from abrasion or chemicals used for sterilization. The thigh should also be draped out in sterile fashion for the option of a fascia lata graft later in the operation.

In patients with a wide laceration over the frontal sinus, the laceration could be incorporated into an incision to access the sinus. However, if the laceration is small or not well-positioned over the fracture requiring repair, a new incision is needed. The coronal incision is ideal as it is situated away from the face and, in most patients, lies behind the hairline.[7,8] Furthermore, the coronal incision allows for exposure and harvesting of a pericranial flap. As shown in Figure 17.4, the coronal incision was used for the example patient. The incision may be made with a scalpel through the epidermis and carried through the galea with the scalpel or needle-point monopolar electrocautery device. Then, the subgaleal plane is dissected with a scalpel, monopolar electrocautery, or Metzenbaum scissors. After the flap is elevated and translated anteriorly, the pericranium is elevated anteriorly with its anterior attachment preserved.

If only the anterior table is displaced, the bone fragments may now be elevated and fixated with a cranial plating set. If there is posterior table displacement or indefinite NFOT competency, the neurosurgeon performs a bifrontal craniotomy, as shown in Figure 17.5. A high-speed burr or perforator is used to create a burr hole on either side of the sagittal sinus. Then, using a Penfield dissector, the dura is separated from the inner table of bone bridging the burr holes. Alternatively, a trough can be made over the sagittal sinus with the burr. To complete the craniotomy, the surgeon uses a high-speed drill with a footplate attachment to make a cut laterally to the superior temporal line, then anteriorly to the orbital rim. If the preexisting fractures do not free the bone flap at this point, the frontal bone is cut just superior to the orbital rim, again with the high-speed drill and footplate or with an osteotome. Taking care to separate the dura from the inner table with a Penfield dissector or periosteal elevator, the bone flap is removed.

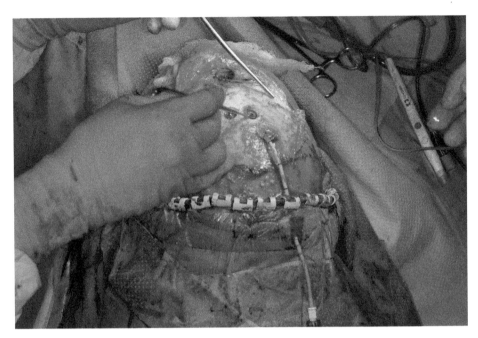

Figure 17.5 Intraoperative photograph of a patient with a frontal sinus fracture. The coronal scalp flap and pericranial graft have been elevated, and burr holes have been created on each side of the frontal sinus. The surgeon is using the Penfield no. 3 instrument to separate the periosteal dura from the inner table of the skull.

Any fractured anterior table fragments may also be removed at this point and fixated to the bone flap in the appropriate positions to restore contour, as shown in Figure 17.6.

If a CSF leak is present, careful intraoperative examination of the dura can reveal the source. Simple dural lacerations may be repaired primarily whereas complex dural lacerations may require repair with a collagen patch or pericranial graft. CSF diversion may reduce the risk of persistent or recurrent CSF leak while the dural repair heals. In patients without intracranial mass lesion or substantial brain edema, this can safely be accomplished with a lumbar drain. However, in patients with traumatic brain injury and brain edema or contusions, an external ventricular drain (EVD) may be placed intraoperatively if not already present. The example patient had a 2 cm dural laceration that was repaired primarily, then covered with a synthetic dural sealant. A right frontal-approach EVD was placed intraoperatively using image guidance.

Next, the NFOT is evaluated. If there is question as to whether the NFOT is obstructed, colored liquid such as fluorescein or methylene blue can be injected into the frontal sinus. Observing the liquid in the middle meatus or nasopharynx indicates patency of NFOT. If there is gross NFOT obstruction or no transmittance of the colored liquid, the frontal sinus is nonfunctional and should be obliterated if the posterior table is intact or cranialized if the posterior table is not intact. The mucosa within the frontal sinus is stripped away, the NOFTs are occluded, and the sinus is packed with fat, temporalis muscle, fascia, or bone chips. Finally, the sinus is sealed with the pericranial graft that was preserved during opening. Alternatively, a surgeon may use a synthetic

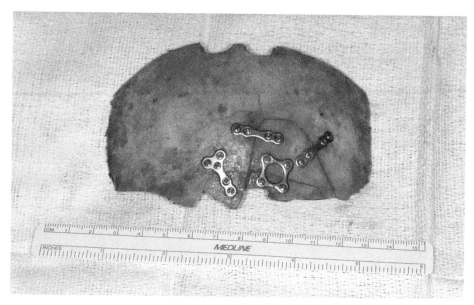

Figure 17.6 Intraoperative photograph. The bifrontal craniotomy flap has been removed, and the fractured anterior table of the frontal sinus has been reduced and fixated with 0.3 mm-thickness titanium neurocranial plates.

graft if preferred or if no serviceable pericranium is intact. Fibrin glue may also be used with the graft to ensure sealing. This process separates the cranium from the external environment.

Once the NFOT functionality has been established and, if necessary, the frontal sinus has undergone obliteration or cranialization, the bone flap may be replaced and fixated with cranial titanium plates (0.3 mm thickness), taking care to approximate the inferior edge of the flap with the orbital rim. Substantial gaps may be covered with split-thickness bone graft or titanium mesh. A subgaleal drain is usually placed, and, in some cases, an epidural drain may be placed before replacing the bone flap, as shown in Figure 17.7. If temporalis was elevated from the superior temporal line, it can be suspended with a cranial fixation plate on top of the muscle or suture tied to a plate that was already placed for bone fixation. Finally, the scalp flap is reapproximated; the galea is closed with 2-0 Vicryl resorbable suture and the skin is closed with staples or sutures, as shown in Figure 17.8.

Pivot Points

- If the anterior table of the frontal sinus is displaced but patency of the NFOT is demonstrated intraoperatively, reduction and fixation of the anterior table should be performed to restore contour, but frontal sinus cranialization is not necessary.
- If NFOT obstruction is observed intraoperatively, then the frontal sinus should be cranialized or obliterated. Attempts to reestablish NFOT drainage are prone to failure.

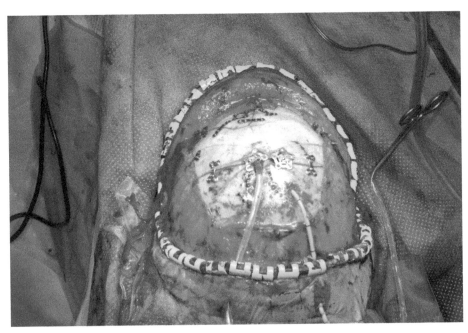

Figure 17.7 Intraoperative photograph of a patient with a frontal sinus fracture. The bone flap has been replaced, and an external ventricular drain and epidural drain exit through the burr holes.

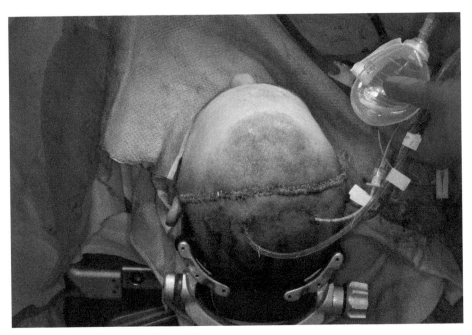

Figure 17.8 Intraoperative photograph of a patient with a frontal sinus fracture. The scalp has been closed with 2-0 Vicryl galeal sutures and skin staples.

- The presence of CSF leakage observed preoperatively or intraoperatively should prompt exploration of the dura and repair of any dural lacerations. In some cases, CSF diversion is needed to lower the risk of recurrent CSF leak while the dural repair heals.

Oral Boards Review: Management Pearls

- Operative intervention for traumatic frontal sinus injuries is predicated on (a) location of the fractures, (b) degree of displacement of the fracture, and the (c) status of the NFOT. Persistent CSF leak is also a strong indication for operative management.
- For those patients who do not undergo surgical repair, clinical and radiographic follow-up is necessary for screening for infectious complications, CSF leak, or development of mucocele/mucopyocele.
- The coronal incision allows for an excellent approach for surgeons to repair frontal sinus fractures. Given its location away from the forehead and behind the hairline, this incision allows for cosmesis and provides the surgical team with the ability to harvest the pericranium, which can be used during surgery to seal off the frontal sinus from the intracranial contents or for purposes of closing traumatic CSF leaks.
- CSF diversion with placement of an EVD or a lumbar drain is a valuable adjunct in patients with dural lacerations to reduce the likelihood of recurrent or persistent CSF leak postoperatively.
- Patency of the NFOT and integrity of the posterior table of the frontal sinus are key determinants in deciding between frontal sinus obliteration or frontal sinus cranialization; regardless, the mucosa within the frontal sinus must be stripped away. The sinus surfaces also need to be drilled because sinus tissue hidden in bone crevices can regrow.

Aftercare

Postoperatively, a head and/or maxillofacial CT may be taken to assess sinus repair and to have as a baseline. Patients should maintain CSF leak precautions, refraining from use of straws, strenuous activity, bearing down, bending over, and blowing the nose. If an EVD or lumbar drain was placed, it should be removed after 3–5 days, depending on security of dural repairs. Forehead sutures should be removed after 5 days, and scalp staples or sutures should be removed after 10–14 days. After suture removal, follow-up with maxillofacial CT at 6 weeks, 3 months, 6 months, then yearly is appropriate to monitor for complications, which may occur years later.[7,8,11,13]

The example patient had been ventilated via an endotracheal (ETT) tube prior to surgery so the ETT was left in place postoperatively. On postoperative day 1 his mental status and respiratory mechanics were sufficient that he was extubated. The EVD was left in place, draining at 0 cm of water above the midbrain for 3 days after surgery, then clamped. With no signs of CSF leak 24 h after the EVD was clamped, it was removed at bedside. Given the patient's substantial frontal brain contusions, he required acute rehabilitation after the frontal sinus fracture repair. The bicoronal incision staples were removed in the rehabilitation facility on postoperative day 14. He was seen in clinic 6 weeks after surgery, at which time he was recovering well without clinical signs of CSF leak, mucocele, or infection, and a head CT demonstrated resolution of pneumocephalus, a cranialized frontal sinus, and improved aeration of the paranasal sinuses.

Complications and Management

Acute complications include CSF leak and infections ranging from soft tissue and sinus infection to intracranial infections including meningitis or brain abscess. CSF leaks can be initially managed with bedrest, head of bed elevation, and CSF diversion. In some cases, reoperation is required to identify the dural defect and repair it. Failure to stop a CSF leak could result in meningitis.

Any sign of infection deep to the skin should be evaluated with a brain MRI with and without contrast, and altered mental status without obvious intracranial abscess should prompt a CSF sample for glucose, protein, cell count, and culture. Superficial soft tissue infections or meningitis alone can be treated with systemic antibiotics, but infections of the sinus or bone or brain abscess or empyema require reoperation for washout and debridement.

Long-term complications include mucocele or mucopyocele, contour deformity, and prominent or exposed hardware. Mucoceles may result from failure to obliterate or cranialize a nonfunctional frontal sinus or failure to remove all the mucosa within the frontal sinus. Mucopyoceles are the most worrisome complication as they can occur years after the injury, and intracranial extension can lead to brain abscesses. Mucoceles and mucopyoceles must be surgically removed to prevent erosion through the bone and intracranial extension, and the sinus must be properly cranialized to prevent recurrence. As swelling resolves and the wound remodels, contour deformities may result if bone fragments are not properly approximated, and hardware such as screws and plates may become palpable or visible under the skin. Exposed hardware must be removed, and, in some cases, local tissue rearrangement or even a soft tissue flap must be used to cover the open area. Surgical revision also may be necessary to correct painful or unsightly prominent hardware or contour deformities.

> ### Oral Boards Review: Complications Pearls
>
> - Early and subacute complications include CSF leak and infections ranging from soft tissue and sinus infection to intracranial infections, inclusive of meningitis and development of brain abscess.
> - Long-term complications include mucocele or mucopyocele, contour deformity, and prominent or exposed hardware.
>   - Mucoceles may result from failure to obliterate or cranialize a nonfunctional frontal sinus or failure to remove all the mucosa within the frontal sinus.
>   - Mucopyoceles are the most worrisome late complication; intracranial extension can lead to brain abscesses.

> • Mucoceles and mucopyoceles must be surgically removed to prevent erosion through the bone and intracranial extension, and the sinus must be properly cranialized to prevent recurrence.

Evidence and Outcomes

There is considerable variability in management strategies described in the literature, especially in regards to sinus preservation versus cranialization or obliteration. Unfortunately, much of the evidence for frontal sinus fracture management is retrospective. One of the largest retrospective reviews by Rodriguez and colleagues (2008) included 857 patients with frontal sinus fractures, 504 of whom underwent surgical management.[9] Patients without NFOT injury had no major complications (i.e., CSF leak, abscess, sinusitis, meningitis, mucocele, persistent pneumocephalus) when observed. Among patients with NFOT injury, those treated with sinus cranialization or obliteration had the lowest complication rates. In a retrospective review of 154 patients, Pollock and colleagues (2013) reported a low complication rate of 6% in patients who had an operation for a frontal sinus fracture, 34 of whom had cranialization of the frontal sinus.[14] The rate of complications was the same for cranialization operations as for other operations, and they attributed the few complications to complete mucosal debridement and NFOT obliteration as well as avoidance of avascular obliteration material. Overall, the data show that patients with NFOT injury have more serious complications but that proper management of NFOT obstruction with technically sound cranialization of the frontal sinus reduces the potential for complications.

Some authors have advocated transnasal, endoscopic, sinus-preserving surgery for frontal sinus fractures, including those with NFOT obstruction. In the otolaryngology literature, a systematic review and a prospective series have demonstrated safety and efficacy of this approach in select patients, mainly those without CSF leak.[15,16] Reported advantages of endoscopic management include lower rates of cosmetic issues, pain, and infections associated with incisions. The advantage of preserving the sinus is the prevention of mucoceles or mucopyoceles forming from reepithelization of a cranialized or obliterated frontal sinus.[15] As technology improves, the management strategies for frontal sinus fractures are evolving.

References and Further Reading

1. Doonquah L, Brown P, Mullings W. Management of frontal sinus fractures. *Oral Maxillofac Surg Clin North Am.* 2012;24(2):265–274, ix. doi:10.1016/j.coms.2012.01.008

2. Stanwix MG, Nam AJ, Manson PN, Mirvis S, Rodriguez ED. Critical computed tomographic diagnostic criteria for frontal sinus fractures. *J Oral Maxillofac Surg.* 2010;68(11):2714–2722. doi:10.1016/j.joms.2010.05.019

3. Oakley GM, Alt JA, Schlosser RJ, Harvey RJ, Orlandi RR. Diagnosis of cerebrospinal fluid rhinorrhea: An evidence-based review with recommendations. *Int Forum Allergy Rhinol.* 2016;6(1):8–16. doi:10.1002/alr.21637

4. Tripathi RC, Millard CB, Tripathi BJ, Noronha A. Tau fraction of transferrin is present in human aqueous humor and is not unique to cerebrospinal fluid. *Experimental Eye Research.* 1990;50(5):541–547. doi:10.1016/0014-4835(90)90043-T

5. Oh J-W, Kim S-H, Whang K. Traumatic cerebrospinal fluid leak: Diagnosis and management. *Korean J Neurotrauma.* 2017;13(2):63. doi:10.13004/kjnt.2017.13.2.63

6. Mathias T, Levy J, Fatakia A, McCoul ED. Contemporary approach to the diagnosis and management of cerebrospinal fluid rhinorrhea. *Ochsner J.* 2016;16(2):136–142.

7. Bitonti, David A., Gentile, Michael A., Respondek, Amy M. Management of frontal sinus fractures. In Kademani D, Tiwana P, eds. *Atlas of Oral and Maxillofacial Surgery- E-Book.* Amsterdam: Elsevier Health Sciences; 2015:816–828.

8. Fattahi, Tirbod. Management of frontal sinus fractures. In Marciani RD, ed. *Oral and Maxillofacial Surgery: Trauma, Surgical Pathology, Temporomandibular Disorders.* Philadelphia: Saunders/Elsevier; 2009:256–269.

9. Rodriguez ED, Stanwix MG, Nam AJ, et al. Twenty-six–year experience treating frontal sinus fractures: A novel algorithm based on anatomical fracture pattern and failure of conventional techniques. *Plast Reconstruct Surg.* 2008;122(6):1850–1866. doi:10.1097/PRS.0b013e31818d58ba

10. Delaney SW. Treatment strategies for frontal sinus anterior table fractures and contour deformities. *J Plast, Reconstruct Aesthet Surg.* 2016;69(8):1037–1045. doi:10.1016/j.bjps.2016.06.006

11. Patel SA, Berens AM, Devarajan K, Whipple ME, Moe KS. Evaluation of a minimally disruptive treatment protocol for frontal sinus fractures. *JAMA Facial Plast Surg.* 2017;19(3):225. doi:10.1001/jamafacial.2016.1769

12. Mundinger G, Borsuk D, Okhah Z, et al. Antibiotics and facial fractures: Evidence-based recommendations compared with experience-based practice. *Craniomaxillofac Trauma Reconstruct.* 2014;08(01):064–078. doi:10.1055/s-0034-1378187

13. Koudstaal MJ, van der Wal KGH, Bijvoet HWC, Vincent AJPE, Poublon RMI. Post-trauma mucocele formation in the frontal sinus: A rationale of follow-up. *Int J Oral Maxillofac Surg.* 2004;33(8):751–754. doi:10.1016/j.ijom.2004.01.019

14. Pollock RA, Hill JL, Davenport DL, Snow DC, Vasconez HC. Cranialization in a cohort of 154 consecutive patients with frontal sinus fractures (1987–2007): Review and update of a compelling procedure in the selected patient. *Ann Plast Surg.* 2013;71(1):54–59. doi:10.1097/SAP.0b013e3182468198

15. Grayson JW, Jeyarajan H, Illing EA, Cho D-Y, Riley KO, Woodworth BA. Changing the surgical dogma in frontal sinus trauma: Transnasal endoscopic repair: Endoscopic repair of frontal sinus trauma. *Int Forum Allergy Rhinol.* 2017;7(5):441–449. doi:10.1002/alr.21897

16. Carter KB, Poetker DM, Rhee JS. Sinus preservation management for frontal sinus fractures in the endoscopic sinus surgery era: A systematic review. *Craniomaxillofac Trauma Reconstr.* 2010;3(3):141–149. doi:10.1055/s-0030-1262957

Penetrating Brain Injuries

Zachary L. Hickman and Konstantinos Margetis

18

Case Presentation

A 20-year-old man with a history of bipolar disorder, recently discharged from a psychiatric hospital, is brought to the emergency department by ambulance following a self-inflicted nail gun injury to the head. The patient is responsive, verbal, and following commands on arrival with an exam notable for mild confusion (Glasgow Coma Scale [GCS] score of 14), a mild left-sided pronator drift, and a small entry wound to the right lateral frontoparietal region of the head with the end of a nail visible. There is no visible egress of brain matter or CSF from the entry wound. There is no apparent exit wound. The patient has no other injuries and no other known medical history.

Questions

1. What are the initial resuscitation steps following penetrating brain injury (PBI)?
2. What is the most appropriate initial imaging modality at this point?
3. What additional imaging modalities should be considered?

Assessment and Planning

PBI may result from missiles (e.g., bullet, shrapnel) or non-missiles (e.g., knife, nail gun). This chapter will focus on the management of PBI resulting from low-velocity or non-missile injuries, while those from gunshots or other high-velocity missiles are discussed in Chapter 19. However, certain principles, including initial trauma resuscitation, concern for associated cerebrovascular injuries, and the risk of posttraumatic seizures (PTS) and infection are common across both major categories of PBI.

Non-missile PBI, with its lower kinetic energy, often has a better prognosis compared to PBI resulting from high-velocity missiles, the latter of which transmits a significant amount of kinetic energy to the surrounding brain tissue, creating temporary and permanent injury cavities. Patients suffering from non-missile PBI are, however, still at significant risk of specific injuries and complications that must be taken into account.

Initial resuscitation of a patient with non-missile PBI should proceed according to the usual ABCs of trauma resuscitation, just as for blunt TBI and missile PBI. Particular attention should be paid to the patient's hemodynamic status and neurological exam, including their GCS score, pupillary and other brainstem reflexes, and any lateralizing signs that may suggest an associated mass lesion, such as an expanding intraparenchymal or extra-axial hematoma. CSF or brain matter may be noted to egress from the entry or exit site from the skull. Additionally, in some cases of PBI, the offending object may be protruding from the patient's skull (e.g., knife, spear gun). In these cases, stabilization of the object following initial resuscitation and before moving the patient (e.g., for imaging scans) is advisable to prevent inadvertent movement or dislodging of the object (Figure 18.1). Stabilization can be attained by applying rolls of gauze or padding around the base of the object as it enters the skull and reinforcing this with tape. In some rare cases, the external portion of the object may need to be carefully cut or trimmed in order for the patient to be safely positioned in a CT scanner. This should be attempted only if absolutely necessary and with extreme caution to avoid any movement of the intracranial portion of the penetrating object. Last, in some cases of nonaccidental PBI, valuable forensic evidence (e.g., fingerprints) may be present on the exposed portion of the object (e.g., knife handle from a stab wound); these can be preserved and contamination avoided by securing a plastic bag over the exposed end of the object and securing it with a rubber band or by covering the object carefully with iodine-impregnated incision (e.g., Ioban) drape.

Noncontrast head CT imaging is the initial imaging study of choice given its rapid acquisition. CT imaging will best demonstrate the tract of the penetrating object, associated intracranial injuries, radiographic evidence of elevated

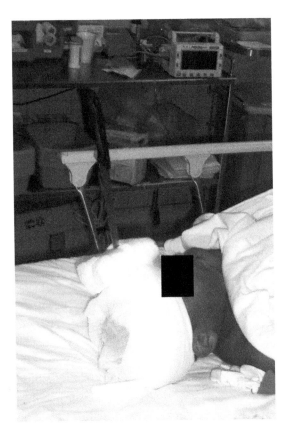

Figure 18.1 Preoperative photograph of a patient with a penetrating stab wound to the head demonstrating temporary stabilization of the penetrating object with gauze rolls and tape prior to patient transport and imaging.

intracranial pressure (ICP), and retained foreign objects in the acute setting. Metallic objects are hyperdense with a characteristic streak artifact, while wooden objects initially have the density of air. If significant anoxic injury has occurred, this may also be visible.

Cerebrovascular imaging, such as a CT angiogram/venogram (CTA/CTV) or catheter-based angiogram, is recommended when the penetrating tract passes through or in close proximity to major arterial or venous intracranial vessels. CTA/CTV allows for rapid evaluation and can be performed at the same time as the initial head CT; however, streak artifact from retained intracranial metallic foreign objects may limit its diagnostic accuracy. A catheter-based angiogram limits streak artifact as well as providing an opportunity for endovascular treatment, if necessary, but may delay emergent life-saving surgical treatment for associated mass lesions or elevated ICP if used for initial screening.

Brain MRI has limited utility in the acute setting following PBI and is generally contraindicated in the presence of retained ferromagnetic foreign bodies, as the magnetic field may cause migration or heating of ferromagnetic objects, resulting in additional direct or thermal injury.

Oral Boards Review: Diagnostic Pearls

- A focused neurological exam (including GCS, pupillary reactivity, and the presence/absence of other brainstem reflexes) following resuscitation is crucial to the diagnosis and management of both missile and non-missile PBI.
  - *Severity of injury and potential for salvage of neurological function.* The neurological exam and improvements with immediate interventions, such as correction of hypotension and hypoxia or mild hyperventilation and hyperosmolar treatment to reduce elevated ICP, helps identify patients with PBI who have potential for salvage of meaningful neurological function.
  - *Signs of herniation that require rapid intervention.* Exam findings such as unilateral/bilateral dilated pupils or a Cushing's response (bradycardia and hypertension) suggest elevated ICP and herniation. Empiric temporizing measures (e.g., mild hyperventilation, hyperosmolar therapy) can be started en route to emergent head imaging.
- Rapid noncontrast head CT imaging is essential to confirm the diagnosis of PBI and to assess the severity of the injury. Poor prognostic findings include bilateral injury, thalamic/brainstem injury, or injuries that cross the midline at the level of the third ventricle or the *zona fatalis* (approximately 4 cm above the dorsum sellae), and evidence of early anoxic brain injury.
  - *Additional penetrating objects.* It is not uncommon to observe additional intracranial penetrating objects (e.g., multiple nails from a nail gun) or penetrating tracts (e.g., knife wound tracts) on head CT imaging that were not identified on the initial physical exam.
- Screening CTA/CTV at the time of the initial head CT is recommended to assess for cerebrovascular injury which may be caused by direct penetrating injury in non-missile PBI.

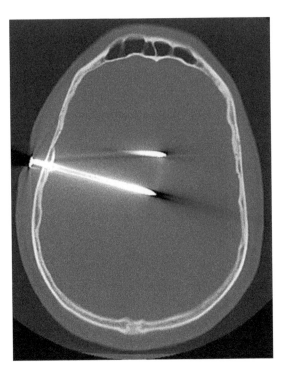

Figure 18.2 Admission axial noncontrast head CT of a 20-year-old man who suffered a self-inflicted nail gun injury.

In the present case, CT imaging demonstrated two nails entering the right lateral frontoparietal region of the skull with the tips just barely crossing midline (Figure 18.2). The end of the first nail had been visualized on physical exam, while the second was completely intracranial and not suspected until imaging was obtained (Figure 18.3).

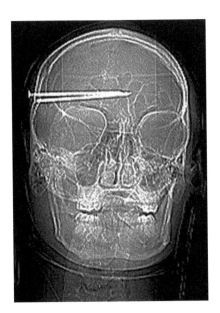

Figure 18.3 Anteroposterior skull x-ray of the patient from Figure 18.2 demonstrating the two penetrating nails.

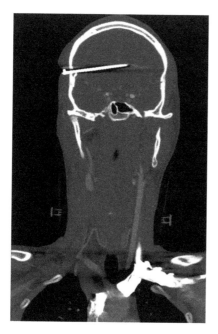

Figure 18.4 Admission coronal CT angiography image of the patient from Figures 18.2 and 18.3 demonstrating one of the nails in close proximity to the right middle cerebral artery (MCA) and anterior cerebral arteries (ACAs), but with no obvious vessel injury.

There was no associated intracranial hematoma (ICH) or other foreign objects noted. A CTA was performed, given the high suspicion for cerebrovascular injury and to aid in operative planning. No vessel injury was seen, but interpretation was limited due to streak artifact (Figure 18.4).

Questions

1. How do these radiological findings influence the management of this patient?
2. What intracranial vessels are most at risk of injury in this case?
3. What are two prophylactic medical treatments that should be routinely instituted following PBI?

Decision Making

The initial decision following PBI is whether or not the patient has potentially salvageable neurological function. Patients with PBI from a high-velocity missile with a poor neurological exam (GCS 3–5, bilaterally nonreactive pupils) often have unfavorable long-term outcomes despite aggressive treatment, while those suffering non-missile PBI often have a significant chance of neurological recovery and a relatively good prognosis. Indications for aggressive intervention in the presence of an initially poor neurological exam include an evacuable mass lesion or other potentially treatable pathology (e.g., acute hydrocephalus from intraventricular hemorrhage [IVH], elevated ICP from focal/diffuse swelling) in combination with a relative paucity of poor prognostic radiographic findings. Given the difficulty in predicting long-term outcomes during initial resuscitation, as well as the imperative for rapid intervention in potentially salvageable patients, it is often advisable to proceed initially with aggressive intervention when radiographic imaging does not demonstrate an obviously fatal injury.

PBI from small or low-velocity objects, such as a stab wound or air gun pellets, may not cause associated mass lesions or a significant amount of cerebral edema. In such cases, surgical intervention is primarily aimed at mitigation of infectious complications through irrigation, limited debridement, dural repair, and wound closure. In some cases, bedside irrigation and closure may be considered if the penetrating object itself is not protruding from the skull (e.g., stab wound with the knife blade no longer present) or the penetrating object is small and not readily surgically accessible (e.g., deep air gun pellets). In many instances, however, the penetrating object may be a source of mass effect itself or in communication with the external environment and necessitate careful surgical removal. Penetrating objects that protrude from the skull (e.g., knife, arrow) should not be removed blindly, but rather under direct vision following craniotomy or craniectomy.

ICP monitor placement should be performed for potentially salvageable patients who are comatose (GCS ≤8) and do not exhibit rapid neurological improvement shortly following resuscitation. Ventriculostomy is the gold standard for ICP monitoring as it allows for therapeutic CSF drainage. If hydrocephalus is not present, a fiberoptic intraparenchymal ICP monitor may be considered instead. The management of elevated ICP and maintenance of adequate cerebral perfusion pressure (CPP) following PBI follows the same principles as for blunt severe traumatic brain injury (sTBI).

In the present case, the patient was noted to have a relatively reassuring neurological exam and radiographic findings consistent with a good prognosis.

Questions

1. What would be an appropriate surgical intervention for this patient?
2. If intracranial vessels are involved on preoperative imaging, what steps should be undertaken to prevent bleeding complications during removal of the penetrating object?

Surgical Procedure

In most cases of low-velocity or non-missile PBI where the patient has a stable neurological exam without an evacuable mass lesion, diffuse cerebral edema, or evidence of elevated ICP, intervention can be performed in an urgent fashion once the patient is hemodynamically stabilized to remove the penetrating object, if necessary, and perform limited superficial debridement, dural repair, and wound closure to reduce the risk of infection. In cases of severe PBI with a mass lesion, cerebral edema, or evidence of elevated ICP, emergent decompressive craniectomy (DC) is advisable if the patient is deemed to be salvageable. In instances where it is unclear whether the patient has salvageable neurological function, it is reasonable to initially manage elevated ICP medically and proceed to definitive surgery if the patient demonstrates neurological improvement with these measures. The potential for significant intraoperative bleeding should be anticipated and adequate amounts of blood products and hemostatic agents should be immediately available for use. This is most pertinent when the penetrating object or missile tract crosses or is in close proximity to known vascular structures. Packed red blood cells (PRBCs), fresh frozen plasma (FFP), cryoprecipitate, and platelets should be ordered and available in ratios according to the hospital massive transfusion protocol (MTP).

For PBI where there is no significant intracranial mass lesion or diffuse cerebral edema requiring emergent decompression, then a plan for craniotomy or craniectomy with removal of a protruding or superficial penetrating object, along with local debridement, dural repair, and wound closure is advocated to mitigate the risk of infection. The scalp incision should be tailored to the surgical objectives and the planned craniotomy or craniectomy. When possible, the incision should not incorporate the entry wound in order to avoid potential wound healing issues, as the edges are often devitalized. Ideally, the entry wound should be debrided and closed separately. An exception is a small entry wound that allows for adequate resection of the devitalized tissue with incorporation into the planned incision and a tensionless closure.

In most instances, a craniotomy or craniectomy is performed centered around the skull entry wound to obtain adequate exposure for object removal, debridement, hemostasis, and dural repair. Involved or fractured bone adjacent to the entry wound is best discarded to reduce postoperative infectious risk. Generally speaking, wide access around the entry site is preferred to allow for adequate visualization of the penetrating object and surrounding brain tissue. Wide access also allows for proximal and distal control of involved intracranial vessels, which should be established prior to object removal to prevent uncontrollable arterial or venous bleeding. Prepping of the ipsilateral neck for temporary carotid artery occlusion should be considered for proximal control of injuries to the main cerebral arteries in the Circle of Willis. Intraoperative cerebral angiography may be particularly useful in these cases.

Debridement is performed with irrigation, gentle suctioning, and careful removal of sizeable superficial bone fragments and foreign objects with forceps. Care should be taken to avoid the temptation to "chase" deep fragments or foreign objects because this increases damage to surrounding brain tissue and risks hemorrhagic complications while providing dubious benefit in reducing infection or long-term seizure incidence. Hemostasis should be obtained and dural repair performed as necessary. In most cases of supratentorial PBI, use of a simple dural substitute onlay is sufficient. Watertight closure is often only necessary when the penetrating injury involves the frontal sinus, mastoid air cells, or the infratentorial fossa, all of which predispose to postoperative CSF leak. A watertight dural closure can be obtained with autograph (e.g., pericranium, tensor fascia lata) or allograft (e.g., bovine pericardium). Pericranium should be harvested some distance from the entry wound to avoid use of potentially contaminated tissue. Titanium mesh is recommended for cranioplasty in most cases due to its inherent resistance to infection compared to other allograft materials. Wound closure should ensure that the edges of the entry wound are adequately debrided and devitalized tissue resected. The scalp may need to be undermined to achieve a tensionless closure. The assistance of plastic surgery is helpful for closure of complex wounds.

DC, either unilateral or bilateral (bifrontal) depending on the injury location, is the surgical treatment of choice for severe PBI with a mass lesion, cerebral edema, and elevated ICP unresponsive to medical management. This is more commonly seen in high-velocity missile injuries, such as a gunshot wound to the head, and is discussed in detail in Chapter 19.

PBI may result in traumatic intracranial pseudoaneurysms that are challenging to repair. These are often best treated via endovascular means. Direct repair during craniotomy or craniectomy may be necessary if there is active bleeding. Options include temporary proximal vessel occlusion followed by direct repair with aneurysm or vessel clips or ligation and sacrifice of distal cerebral vessels, if necessary.

Injury to dural venous sinuses may be managed by leaving an island of bone over the injury site to allow for dural tack-up stitches to control epidural bleeding. Sinus ligation may occasionally be needed; this can often be performed without untoward complication in the anterior one-third of the superior sagittal sinus and the nondominant transverse or sigmoid sinus. Alternatively, bleeding from dural sinus injuries will frequently cease following tamponade with absorbable hemostatic sponges augmented with fibrin glue or sealant. Attempts to remove penetrating bone or foreign objects from a dural venous sinus injury should generally be avoided due to the risk of profuse bleeding that may be challenging to control. In some cases, injuries may cause partial sinus occlusion and predispose to venous sinus thrombosis and elevated ICP. Since therapeutic anticoagulation for sinus thrombosis is inherently risky following PBI, there may be a need for direct sinus repair. This can be achieved through temporary sinus occlusion followed by repair of the sinus injury with dural autograft or allograft, muscle plug, or temporalis fascia. A common method is to fold and tack a leaflet of nearby dura over the injury site. Application of fibrin glue or sealant can help reinforce the repair.

In the present case, the patient underwent an urgent right frontoparietal craniotomy with wide exposure around the penetrating nails. Preoperative CTA demonstrated no vessel injury; however, proximal and distal vessel control was established prior to removal to avoid bleeding complications. The nails were carefully removed under direct visualization. The local brain tissue was superficially debrided, hemostasis obtained, and the dura closed. The portion of bone immediately around the entry site was craniectomized and the defect repaired with a titanium mesh cranioplasty. The scalp incision was closed in the usual fashion and the nail entry sites debrided and closed separately.

Oral Boards Review: Management Pearls

- Patients presenting with a good neurological exam and without need for emergent cerebral decompression and evacuation of mass lesions should undergo surgical intervention in most cases for removal of protruding or exposed foreign objects, superficial debridement, dural repair, and wound closure to reduce the risk of CSF leak and infection.
- Penetrating foreign objects should only be removed under direct visualization. Wide exposure is recommended, as is proximal and distal vascular control if a cerebrovascular injury is known or suspected. Intraoperative neuroendovascular approaches may be useful to mitigate bleeding from vessels where direct proximal control is difficult.
- Rapid cerebral decompression and evacuation of mass lesions for control of elevated ICP and prevention of herniation in patients with salvageable

neurological function is warranted to improve survival and functional outcome. Comatose PBI patients (GCS ≤ 8) should have ICP/CPP monitored and managed following similar principles as for blunt sTBI.

- Seizure prophylaxis should be routinely instituted following PBI to reduce the risk of early PTS.
- Most neurosurgeons advocate for aggressive empiric broad-spectrum antibiotic prophylaxis following PBI.

Pivot Points

- Development of fulminant cerebral edema during surgery should prompt additional maneuvers to maximize decompression and reduce ICP, including extension of the craniectomy, elevation of the head, mild hyperventilation, hyperosmolar therapy, placement of an external ventricular drain, and partial frontal or temporal lobectomy, as necessary.
- Profuse bleeding from injured cerebral blood vessels should be controlled expeditiously to prevent development of disseminated intravascular coagulation (DIC), coagulopathy, and exsanguination. Appropriate equipment and instruments should be immediately available in the event that direct vessel occlusion is required, including the operating microscope and aneurysm or vessel clips. Surgical planning should allow for proximal and distal control of suspected injured vessels.
- Extensive intraoperative blood loss should be anticipated and trigger activation of the hospital MTP if encountered. Replacement of coagulation factors and platelets is crucial to prevent DIC. Adjuncts such as prothrombin complex concentrate (PCC) or tranexamic acid (TXA) may be useful if coagulopathy develops.

Aftercare

Patients with PBI should be treated with prophylactic antibiotics to reduce the risk of infection from contaminated foreign objects. The specific antibiotic agents and duration of treatment is a controversial issue; the length of treatment extends up to 6 weeks in some protocols. We advocate for at least 5–7 days of empiric broad-spectrum antibiotics, typically a combination of intravenous vancomycin, cefepime, and metronidazole. Use of topical vancomycin powder, which has been shown to reduce the risk of postsurgical infections in multiple types of elective cranial and spine surgeries, can be considered as an adjunct during surgery for PBI to prevent local infection.

Antiepileptic drugs (AEDs) should be administered following PBI and continued for at least 7 days to reduce the incidence of early PTS. There is controversy regarding the duration of the treatment, but extrapolation from blunt sTBI guidelines suggests that a 7-day course may be sufficient. However, the relatively high incidence of late-onset

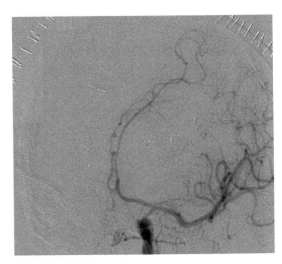

Figure 18.5 Cerebral angiogram of a 24-year-old patient 1 week following penetrating brain injury demonstrating delayed formation of a two small left callosomarginal artery pseudoaneurysms. This patient's initial screening CT angiogram had demonstrated no vessel injury. Both pseudoaneurysms were successfully treated via endovascular embolization.

seizures and posttraumatic epilepsy following PBI, coupled with the favorable side-effect profiles of newer AEDs, has resulted in a trend toward prolonged AED administration.

Serial imaging should be followed to assess for interval evolution or resolution of intracranial hemorrhages and edema, intracranial abscess formation, and delayed posttraumatic hydrocephalus.

If there is high suspicion of cerebrovascular injury, but initial vascular imaging is negative, a repeat CT or cerebral angiogram should be considered approximately 7–10 days following PBI to detect delayed development of pseudoaneurysm, arterial dissection, venous sinus thrombosis, or arteriovenous fistula (Figure 18.5). These may be amenable to endovascular or open treatment (pseudoaneurysms, fistulas) or require antithrombotic medications (dissection, sinus thrombosis).

Following severe PBI, the principles of ICP/CPP management for severe TBI should be followed, with escalation of treatment in a tiered fashion.

Complications and Management

Infection is a well-known complication of PBI. Retained contaminated foreign bodies, CSF leak, and wound healing issues strongly predispose to this complication. Debridement and drainage of intracranial abscesses should be performed expeditiously.

Hydrocephalus can develop in an acute or delayed fashion, particularly in the setting of IVH.

Delayed intracranial hemorrhage or infarction can develop from cerebrovascular injury. Cerebral angiogram (CT or catheter-based) is indicated in such settings.

Cerebral vasospasm may develop secondary to traumatic subarachnoid hemorrhage or the cavitation shock wave from high-velocity missiles. Serial transcranial Doppler ultrasonography and CTA can help diagnose vasospasm and allow for early initiation of treatment before clinical deterioration.

Venous sinus thrombosis can cause elevated ICP.

Delayed CSF leak may develop. Early CSF leaks may respond to temporary CSF diversion via external ventricular or lumbar drainage. Delayed CSF leaks are unlikely to respond to conservative therapy due to fistula formation and may require endoscopic or open surgery to repair. The CSF leak site may occur distant to the entry/exit wound via a "blow out" mechanism, due to formation of the temporary cavity from high-velocity missiles.

Delayed attempts to remove deep-seated bone or missile fragments may be indicated if these obstruct CSF flow, form a nidus for intracranial abscess, or for a migrating fragment that causes additional delayed injury. The presence of heavy metals in some foreign objects (lead in some bullets) may cause delayed toxicity, though this is quite rare.

PTS and epilepsy are not uncommon following PBI. Resumption of AEDs or prolonged administration may be necessary. EEG and consultation with neurology is helpful in these circumstances.

Oral Boards Review: Complications Pearls

- Postoperative cerebral swelling and the need for continued aggressive ICP/CPP management should be expected following PBI, particularly from high-velocity missiles.
- Infection and seizures are relatively common following PBI and should be anticipated and managed prophylactically.
- Development of delayed intracranial abscess should be managed in an urgent fashion with abscess drainage, additional debridement of contaminated bone/missile fragments, and wound washout.

Evidence and Outcomes

Predictors for poor outcome following PBI include (1) older age, (2) low initial GCS (GCS 3–5), (3) bilateral dilated/fixed pupils, (4) hypotension, (5) respiratory depression, (6) coagulopathy, (7) suicide attempt, (8) high-velocity missile injury, (9) perforating ("through-and-through") injury, (10) transventricular injury, (11) intraventricular or subarachnoid hemorrhage, (12) basal cistern effacement, and (13) elevated ICP.

Further Reading

Guidelines for the management of penetrating brain injury. *J Trauma*. 2001 Aug;51(2)(Suppl):S1–S43.

Prognosis in penetrating brain injury. *J Trauma*. 2001 Aug;51(2)(Suppl):S44–S86.

Bodanapally UK, Saksobhavivat N, Shanmuganathan K, Aarabi B, Roy AK. Arterial injuries after penetrating brain injury in civilians: Risk factors on admission head computed tomography. *J Neurosurg*. 2015 Jan;122(1):219–26. http://www.ncbi.nlm.nih.gov/pubmed/25361486

Kazim SF, Shamim MS, Tahir MZ, Enam SA, Waheed S. Management of penetrating brain injury. *J Emerg Trauma Shock*. 2011 Jul;4(3):395–402. http://www.ncbi.nlm.nih.gov/pubmed/21887033

Management of Gunshot Wounds to the Head

Bizhan Aarabi

19

Case Presentation

Attempting suicide, a 37-year-old woman shot herself in the mouth; within 1 h she was airlifted to the trauma resuscitation unit (TRU), sedated, and intubated. In the TRU, her oral cavity was full of clot; her blood pressure was 140/90, pulse rate 55. She was unconscious (Glasgow Coma Scale [GCS] score = 5, motor score 3). Her left pupil was 5 mm and nonreactive to light with an almost frozen left eye. Right pupil was 4 mm in diameter and reactive to light. Right corneal reflex was present, and cold caloric stimulation induced tonic deviation of the right eye to the right side. She did not move her right arm and right leg to painful stimuli but flexed her left arm forcefully.

Questions

1. What is your clinical impression?
2. What imaging modalities best aid in management?
3. What anatomical regions of the intracranial compartments would you study in imaging studies?
4. What is the most appropriate timing for imaging studies and treatment?

Assessment and Planning

What we now know about the standard management of gunshot wounds to the head (GSWH) has been learned across a time span of more than 100 years, during World Wars I and II, the Korean and Vietnam campaigns, and regional conflicts in the Middle East and Balkans.[1–8] GSWH are inherently open wounds with the possibility of deep brain infections if not managed appropriately. Retained bone or metal fragments (Figure 19.1B,D,E) are prime suspects for causing deep brain abscesses, subdural and epidural empyema, or meningitis.[9–11] Projectiles may traverse air sinuses upon entering the intracranial cavity, thus violating the subarachnoid space, cisterns, or the ventricular system (Figure 19.1B,C,F). Because the brain is a huge vascular structure, bone or metal fragments traversing across cerebral tissue might cause intracerebral hematomas (ICH) (Figure 19.1E,F) and/or traumatic intracranial aneurysms (TICA) (Figure 19.2).[15,16,18,19] Do we have to worry about minute retained bone fragments (Figure 19.1A,B)?[10,20 21] How important is it to repair a violated or torn dura matter to prevent CSF leakage (Figure 19.1B,C,D,F)?[11,12,24,25]

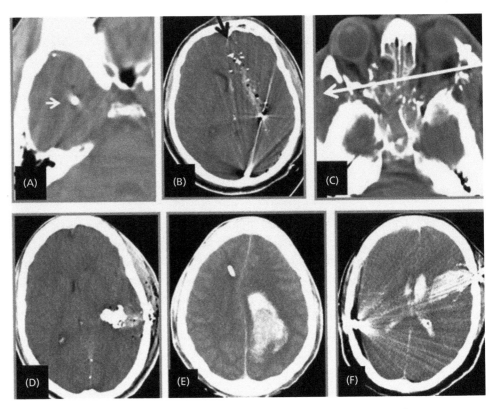

Figure 19.1 Gunshot wound to the head possibilities depicted in six different scenarios. (A) Penetration of a pellet striking the squamous portion of right temporal fossa and residing in brain without causing intracerebral hematoma and destruction of brain parenchyma. (B) Bullet penetrated the frontal bone, frontal sinus, and left hemisphere and finally resided in the left occipital lobe with retained bone and metal fragments in the bullet tract. (C) A single bullet entered the left orbital cavity and broke into the ethmoid sinuses and skull base, finally exiting from the right orbital wall. (D) Penetrating injury of the left parietal bone with a large number of retained bone fragments and brain tissue destruction. (E) Penetrating brain injury of left parietal bone causing left parietal intracerebral hematoma. (F) Perforating and fatal brain injury by a bullet entering the right fronto–parietal region and crossing the sagittal axial and coronal planes into the central gray matter and the ventricular system, eventually exiting through the left frontal bone. There are intracerebral and intraventricular hematomas.

Oral Boards Review: Diagnostic Pearls

- Minute pellets or retained bone fragments seem to be innocuous, rarely causing serious infections.[12]
- Fragments that traverse frontal or ethmoid sinuses need meticulous dural repair.[9,11]
- Significant quantities of superficial retained bone fragments need to be debrided.[9,13,14]
- Intracerebral hematomas must be studied with CTA to rule out TICA.[15–19]

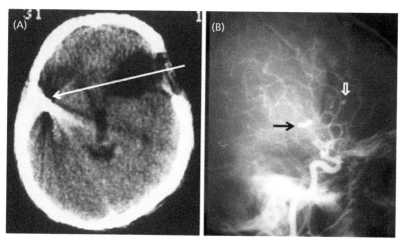

Figure 19.2 Penetrating brain injury with bullet penetrating the left pterional region, causing a pericallosal anterior cerebral artery (ACA) traumatic aneurysm. The projectile was eventually stopped by the opposite inner table of skull. This aneurysm was discovered during the postoperative course when the patient was studied by digital subtraction angiography.

- Moribund patients with GCS 3–5, fixed and dilated pupils, and a fragment traversing sagittal or coronal compartments of the brain should be treated nonoperatively.[22,23]

Questions

1. How do clinical and radiological findings influence surgical planning?
2. What is the most appropriate timing for intervention in this patient?
3. What is the best surgical technique to manage open wounds, prevent CSF leakage, and manage TICA?

The neurosurgeon dealing with GSWH should be aware of a few fundamental realities: (1) close to 90% of patients with GSWH die at the scene; therefore, we have to do our best to save a few through early wound debridement and repair of CSF leaks; (2) retained bone fragments are contaminated and should be removed from the superficial part of the tract during debridement; (3) vascular injuries need to be repaired early and be eliminated either by endovascular means or surgical intervention.

Oral Board Review: Management Pearls

- Open wounds through air sinuses should be taken seriously because of torn dura.
- Neurosurgeons, plastic surgeons, oromaxillofacial surgeons, and ENT surgeons should work together to definitively repair a torn and macerated scalp wound to prevent CSF leakage and meningitis.

- Patients with fragments traversing the region of the middle cerebral and anterior cerebral arteries (MCA, ACA) and crossing the sagittal, axial, or coronal planes with or without ICH should have CT angiography to rule out dormant aneurysms.
- Transventricular injuries are especially prone to CSF leak from the scalp.

Decision Making

Surgical Procedure

Before surgery, one needs to review the imaging studies and look for the following:

1. What is the course of the bullet? Is the tract peripheral, or does it traverse the central gray?
2. Is there stellate fracture of the skull indicating a temporary cavity?
3. Is there ICH near the MCA or ACA indicating the possibility of TICAs?
4. Is there torn and macerated scalp?
5. Is there massive tissue destruction?

Patients with small fragment injuries who are conscious and in whom the fragments are not associated with large ICH or crossing of major vascular structures should be managed by simple wound debridement without craniectomy or craniotomy (Figure 19.3). Experience has proved that fragments are sterile, do not cause abscess, and are minute and do not need removal. Guidelines for the prognosis and management of penetrating head injury agrees with this concept.[26] Small fragments crossing the candelabra of the MCA or with an entrance near the pterion should be examined with CTA to rule out vascular lesions.

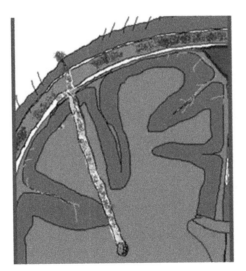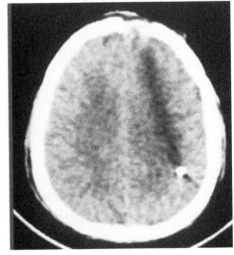

Figure 19.3 The CT image and the drawing show a shell fragment crossing the centrum semiovale without intracerebral hematoma or significant destruction of the cerebral mantle.

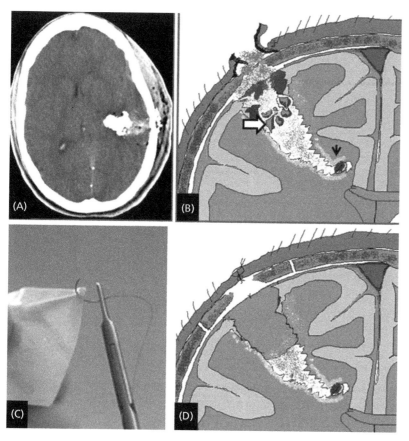

Figure 19.4 Preoperative (A,B) and postoperative (D) schematic and axial CT views of a patient with penetrating injury of left parietal region (A). The CT (A) and drawing (B) show massive retained bone fragments. Figure C shows a graft implant and the drawing in figure D shows a complete watertight closure of the dura and skin following debridement.

Patients with tangential, penetrating, or perforating injuries with significant destruction of brain and retained bone fragments but who have a chance of acceptable outcome must have radical surgery.[26] These patients need conventional craniotomy, debridement of the superficial bone and pulped brain, grafting of the dura, and watertight closure of the scalp and dura. Treatment should comprise other surgical teams, including plastic, ENT, and oromaxillofacial surgeons (Figure 19.4). Following debridement, intracranial pressure (ICP) monitoring (Figure 19.5) will indicate whether decompressive craniectomy and expansive duraplasty are needed.

Penetrating injuries crossing the frontal, ethmoid, and sphenoid sinuses or mastoid air cells are especially dangerous in predisposing patients to CSF leaks and deep intracranial infections.[27–29] Figure 19.6 depicts the clinical course of the case presented in this chapter. The projectile penetrated the skull base (Figure 19.6A,B) and lacerated the dura, crossing into the left frontal lobe, striking the inner table, and ricocheting toward the posterior parietal region (Figure 19.6A). She had an acute subdural hematoma causing a significant shift of the midline structures from left to right (Figure 19.6C). Because of penetration into the territory of the ACA and MCA, she

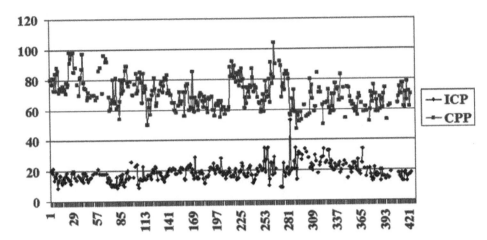

Figure 19.5 Graph indicating intracranial pressure (ICP) monitoring during the critical care management course of the patient described in Figure 19.4 over at least 15 days following primary debridement. The patient needed secondary decompressive craniectomy around day 10 for control of ICP.

underwent a CTA (Figure 19.6A), which did not indicate dormant traumatic vascular injuries. Through a left fronto-parieto-temporal craniotomy, the subdural hematoma was evacuated, the dollar-size dural defect was grafted, and an expansive duraplasty was performed (Figure 19.6D,E).[3,30] The patient had ICP monitoring and maximum medical management. Three months following injury, she had a left fronto-parieto-temporal cranioplasty (Figure 19.6F). Six months after admission, the patient was conscious, alert, blind in the left eye, and with only slight weakness of the right distal lower extremity.

Pivot Points

- Always have help from plastic, oromaxillofacial, and ENT surgeons if you can't repair the scalp yourself.
- Be prepared for extensive dural laceration repair at the skull base.
- Beware of CSF leakage from skull base wounds: they don't heal, and you may need lumbar drainage for a few days.
- Do not explore ICH without CT angiography.

Aftercare

Patients with GSWH need to be on anticonvulsants for longer than a week if their hospital course during the first week of hospitalization is complicated by seizures. If fragmented skull is contaminated, use an allograft implant for cranioplasty. If there is a new CSF leak, re-explore and repair again. If there are more than a few small retained bone fragments, order a CT with contrast in 4–6 weeks to rule out abscess.

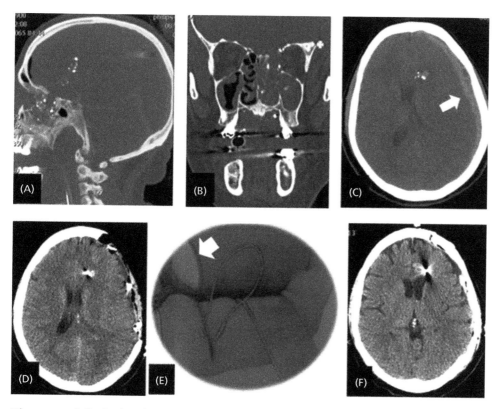

Figure 19.6 Sagittal and coronal CT scan bone windows (A,B), axial brain windows (C,D,F), and schematic view from skull base indicating repair of dura (E).

Figures A, B, C: Admission CT views with bullet penetrating the skull base and acute subdural hematoma on the left side.

Figure D: Postoperative view following decompressive craniectomy.

Figure E: Repair of skull base dura.

Figure F: CT scan was obtained following cranioplasty 3 months after trauma.

Oral Boards Review: Complication Pearls

- In the case of a new CSF leak and meningitis, the dural tear needs to be repaired again.
- Over long-term follow-up, nearly 50% of patients with GSWH become epileptic and need consultation with and management by a neurologist.
- Delayed traumatic ICH (DTICH) is usually due to TICA and must be evaluated by CT angiography or digital subtraction angiography (DSA) and managed appropriately by endovascular or surgical means.

Additional Reading

1. Aarabi B. Surgical outcome in 435 patients who sustained missile head wounds during the Iran-Iraq War. *Neurosurgery.* Nov 1990;27(5):692–695; discussion, 695.

2. Ascroft P. Treatment of head wounds due to missiles. Analysis of 500 cases. *Lancet (London, England).* 1943;2:211–218.

3. Bell RS, Mossop CM, Dirks MS, et al. Early decompressive craniectomy for severe penetrating and closed head injury during wartime. *Neurosurg Focus.* May 2010;28(5):E1.

4. Carey ME, Young HF, Mathis JL. The neurosurgical treatment of craniocerebral missile wounds in Vietnam. *Surg Gynecol Obstet.* Sep 1972;135(3):386–389.

5. Cushing H. A study of a series of wounds involving the brain and its enveloping structures. *Br J Surg.* 1918;5:558–684.

6. Levi L, Linn S, Feinsod M. Penetrating craniocerebral injuries in civilians. *Br J Neurosurg.* 1991;5(3):241–247.

7. Meirowsky AM, Harsh GR. The surgical management of cerebritis complicating penetrating wounds of the brain. *J Neurosurg.* Jul 1953;10(4):373–379.

8. Vrankovic D, Hecimovic I, Splavski B, Dmitrovic B. Management of missile wounds of the cerebral dura mater: Experience with 69 cases. *Neurochirurgia (Stuttg).* Sep 1992;35(5):150–155.

9. Aarabi B, Taghipour M, Alibaii E, Kamgarpour A. Central nervous system infections after military missile head wounds. *Neurosurgery.* Mar 1998;42(3):500–507; discussion 507-509.

10. Carey ME, Young HF, Rish BL, Mathis JL. Follow-up study of 103 American soldiers who sustained a brain wound in Vietnam. *J Neurosurg.* Nov 1974;41(5):542–549.

11. Meirowsky AM, Caveness WF, Dillon JD, et al. Cerebrospinal fluid fistulas complicating missile wounds of the brain. *J Neurosurg.* Jan 1981;54(1):44–48.

12. Aarabi B. Causes of infections in penetrating head wounds in the Iran-Iraq War. *Neurosurgery.* Dec 1989;25(6):923–926.

13. Campbell EH, Jr., Martin J. Cerebral fungus following penetrating wounds. *Surgery.* May 1946;19:748–755.

14. Levi L, Borovich B, Guilburd JN, et al. Wartime neurosurgical experience in Lebanon, 1982-85. II: Closed craniocerebral injuries. *Isr J Med Sci.* Oct 1990;26(10):555–558.

15. Aarabi B. Management of traumatic aneurysms caused by high-velocity missile head wounds. *Neurosurg Clin N Am.* Oct 1995;6(4):775–797.

16. Amirjamshidi A, Abbassioun K, Rahmat H. Traumatic aneurysms and arteriovenous fistulas of the extracranial vessels in war injuries. *Surg Neurol.* Feb 2000;53(2):136–145.

17. Bell RS, Vo AH, Roberts R, Wanebo J, Armonda RA. Wartime traumatic aneurysms: Acute presentation, diagnosis, and multimodal treatment of 64 craniocervical arterial injuries. *Neurosurgery.* Jan 2010;66(1):66–79; discussion 79.

18. Haddad FS, Haddad GF, Taha J. Traumatic intracranial aneurysms caused by missiles: Their presentation and management. *Neurosurgery.* Jan 1991;28(1):1–7.

19. Jinkins JR, Dadsetan MR, Sener RN, Desai S, Williams RG. Value of acute-phase angiography in the detection of vascular injuries caused by gunshot wounds to the head: Analysis of 12 cases. *Am J Roentgenol.* Aug 1992;159(2):365–368.

20. Aarabi B. Comparative study of bacteriological contamination between primary and secondary exploration of missile head wounds. *Neurosurgery.* Apr 1987;20(4):610–616.

21. Carey ME. Learning from traditional combat mortality and morbidity data used in the evaluation of combat medical care. *Mil Med.* Jan 1987;152(1):6–13.

22. Aarabi B, Tofighi B, Kufera J, et al. Predictors of outcome in civilian gunshot wounds to the head. Paper presented at the Annual Meeting of the Congress of Neurological Surgeons (CNS) 2013; San Francisco, CA, USA.

23. Kaufman HH, Levy ML, Stone JL, et al. Patients with Glasgow Coma Scale scores 3, 4, 5 after gunshot wounds to the brain. *Neurosurg Clin N Am*. Oct 1995;6(4):701–714.

24. Gonul E, Erdogan E, Tasar M, et al. Penetrating orbitocranial gunshot injuries. *Surg Neurol*. Jan 2005;63(1):24–30; discussion, 31.

25. Velanovich V. A meta-analysis of prophylactic antibiotics in head and neck surgery. *Plast Reconstr Surg*. Mar 1991;87(3):429–434; discussion, 435.

26. Aarabi B, Alden B, Chesnut RM, al. e. Management and prognosis of penetrating brain injury. *J Trauma*. 2001;51(Suppl):S1–S85.

27. Aarabi B, Leibrock LG. Neurosurgical approaches to cerebrospinal fluid rhinorrhea. *ENT J*. Jul 1992;71(7):300–305.

28. Arendall RE, Meirowsky AM. Air sinus wounds: An analysis of 163 consecutive cases incurred in the Korean War, 1950–1952. *Neurosurgery*. Oct 1983;13(4):377–380.

29. Cairns H. Injuries of the frontal and ethmoidal sinuses with special reference to cerebrospinal rhinorrhoea and aerocele. *J Laryng*. 1937;52.

30. Cooper DJ, Rosenfeld JV, Murray L, et al. Decompressive craniectomy in diffuse traumatic brain injury. *N Engl J Med*. Apr 21 2011;364(16):1493–1502.

Management of Complex Scalp Injuries

Thana N. Theofanis and Patrick Greaney

20

Case Presentation

A 28-year-old man presents to the trauma bay having suffered a gunshot wound to the skull. He was driving around a car and bystanders report they heard firing, otherwise details of the incident are unknown.

He is maintaining his airway. The patient is opening his eyes to pain, mumbling incomprehensible sounds, and localizing to pain.

There was a right frontal entry point and a left frontal exit point. It appears that the bullet traversed through the skull and was lodged in the subcutaneous tissue over the left maxillary region. There was exposed herniated brain to the right frontal entry point. Head CT of the patient is shown in Figure 20.1.

Questions

1. How should this patient be triaged? What is his Glasgow Coma Scale (GCS) score? What type of unit should the patient be admitted to?
2. What are key aspects of the history and physical in this patient?
3. What additional imaging, if any, should be obtained?
4. What is your working diagnosis?

Assessment and Planning

An appreciation for the complexity and implications of a scalp laceration hinges on a solid understanding of the anatomy of the scalp and calvaria; therefore we will provide a brief review. The scalp is comprised of five layers: skin, subcutaneous fat, galea aponeurotica, loose areolar tissue, and pericranium. The galea continues anteriorly as the frontal muscle, posteriorly as the occipital muscle, and laterally is continuous with the temporoparietal fascia. Vascular supply to the scalp is comprised of the following pairs of vessels: supratrochlear, supraorbital, superficial temporal, posterior auricular and occipital arteries, and associated draining veins. While the supratrochlear and supraorbital arteries arise from the ophthalmic artery (first branch of internal carotid artery [ICA]), the others listed are all external carotid artery branches. The nerve supply to the scalp is comprised of the following pairs of nerves: supratrochlear (V1), supraorbital (V1), zygomaticotemporal (V2), auriculotemporal (V3), lesser occipital (C2–C3), and greater occipital (C2). The calvarium contains three layers: outer table, diploic space, and inner table. Children reach complete calvarial growth by around the age of 7 years.

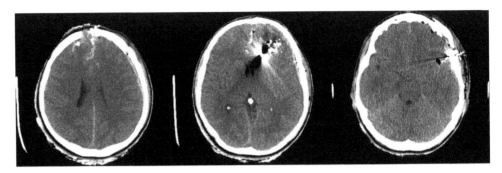

Figure 20.1 Series of axial noncontrast CT head scans of patient who suffered a gunshot wound to the head. There was a right frontal entry point, and the bullet traversed the brain parenchyma and exited to become embedded in the soft tissues of the left maxillary region.

A surgical team should perform initial inspection of a complex scalp laceration, including the surrounding tissues and any previous scalp incisions. The patient should receive appropriate analgesia to enable the team to examine the extent of the injury. If the surgeon needs to touch the skin, this should be done with sterile gloves and delicate handling of the injured tissue. Additionally, if the injury cannot be visualized secondary to hair in the surgical site, the team should be prepared to shave the hair around the injury. The inspection of the scalp wound should be done in a setting with ample lighting and care. The incision should be copiously irrigated with saline and cleaned with a topical antiseptic such as Betadine or ChloraPrep solution.

Due to the robust blood supply to the scalp, complex lacerations can sometimes be a source of significant blood loss. If this is the case, it is of utmost importance that this be recognized and the incision be closed quickly with staples or the head wrapped to tamponade the bleeding until the patient is stable. The ABC's of an initial trauma survey should not be forgotten. A patient with a complex scalp laceration is likely to have other injuries on his or her face and body. The management of a complex scalp laceration will often not be the first priority unless it is associated with open/depressed skull fracture and additional underlying brain traumatic injury as well.

In the case presented here, the patient has a GCS score of 9 and does not meet definitive criteria for intubation at present but should be watched diligently for any signs of deterioration. In this case, a moist dressing should be applied to the wound as the primary and secondary trauma surveys take place.

Oral Boards Review: Diagnostic Pearls

- The scalp is composed of five layers and has a robust vascular supply, which can make scalp wounds a source of significant blood loss.
- It is vital for the physician to examine, clean, and temporarily close or pack a complex scalp wound that does not require immediate repair. If permanent repair is occurring at the bedside, the clinician should be experienced in surgical tissue handling and in closing wounds in a sterile and controlled fashion.

Decision Making

When inspecting the scalp laceration, the surgeon should consider a number of factors. First, is the scalp wound partial thickness or full thickness in depth? Partial-thickness scalp lacerations may be closed with a simple dissolvable suture or staples at the bed-side or occasionally be allowed to heal by secondary intention in selected cases. This is an option that should be preferentially considered in patients who are at high-risk for surgical reconstruction in the operating room. Second, it is important to pay attention to the shape of the laceration with respect to its location on the scalp and pattern of blood supply. Third, one must consider the mechanism of injury: Was this a blunt penetrating trauma that made a clean cut, such as a knife wound? Or did the patient sustain a thermal or electrical burn that caused a significant amount of tissue to be nonviable? Also, in cases such as a gunshot wound, the surgical team must be aware of the location of any foreign bodies (i.e., bullet fragments) and how these will be addressed and ultimately removed if possible.

Preoperative imaging should include a noncontrast head CT at minimum. Often, an MRI is not indicated. A Doppler machine should be available for assessing arterial supply to a potential flap, and, if a free flap is even a consideration, a microscope and micro instruments should be in the operating room and available immediately if they are needed.

Other important considerations include inspecting the pericranium to see if it is intact. The pericranium is a robustly vascular layer atop the calvarium and can be crucial to repairs in some cases. Additionally, if there is an underlying skull fracture, neurosurgical assistance may be required for potential craniotomy/craniectomy with possible cranioplasty or even inspection of underlying dura. If the patient is critically ill from other systemic trauma, the complex scalp laceration may be temporarily closed at the bedside, and the patient can be taken to the operating room at a later time for a repair when medically stable.

In the case presented at the beginning of this chapter, the patient has exposed and herniated brain, which will require urgent surgical attention. Since the patient lacked any other serious systemic injuries and was hemodynamically stable, the decision was made to take the patient to the operating room the night he arrived to the trauma bay.

Questions

1. Will surgery entail a simple closure or staged closure?
2. If there is an underlying skull fracture, how will this be addressed? Do you need to perform a craniotomy/craniectomy?
3. How will you be prepared to deal with damaged dura or a CSF leak? A fracture/injury involving the frontal sinus? A vessel injury or contusion of the brain parenchyma?

Surgical Procedure

Generally speaking, patients with full-thickness scalp wounds should undergo some form of reconstructive surgery. Options for surgical closure of complex scalp lacerations include primary closure, skin grafts, tissue expansion, local flaps, regional flaps, and free flaps. The primary goal of surgery is ultimately to achieve closure of the defect, whether it be in an immediate or delayed fashion. A secondary goal is to maintain all motor and sensory functions of the scalp and face. Finally, the surgeon should always keep cosmesis in mind, although this is certainly not necessarily the top priority in the setting of scalp/ facial trauma. In general, incisions should be placed behind the hairline and the temporalis muscle should be spared and left intact when possible.

Primary closure is an excellent option for smaller scalp wounds and lacerations, typically 3 cm or less. The scalp is relatively inelastic. Therefore, to assist with primary closure, the surgeon may need to circumferentially undermine the surrounding tissue in order to ease the process of closing the skin primarily. Occasionally, scoring of the galea itself is useful to release tension and facilitate closure. Options for closing the skin in this way include a 2-0 Vicryl layer for the galea, followed by a Monocryl subcuticular or staples on the skin. Another excellent but often underutilized stitch in the setting of trauma is the vertical mattress nylon suture, which can provide an excellent bolster to reapproximate the skin edges under minimal tension. If primary closure is used, the surgeon must pay attention to the quality of the skin edges that are being brought together: a poorly vascularized skin edge or one that has undergone repeated trauma is unlikely to heal and may need to be ellipsed/excised out. Furthermore, an incision under considerable tension often results in wound breakdown.

Skin grafts, full- or split-thickness, are an option when primary closure is not able to be accomplished. A skin graft requires a vascularized wound base, thus it is imperative that at the very least a layer of healthy, intact pericranium lies below the area of the planned graft. In some cases, synthetic options, such as an Integra skin substitute, may be a suitable option. Integra is a bi-layered skin substitute made of a silicone membrane (functioning as the "epidermal layer") and collagen. After application and a variable period of several weeks required for vascularization of the graft, the superficial silicone layer is then removed and a thin split-thickness skin graft is applied over the neodermal bed. Disadvantages of the Integra graft are that it typically requires multiple procedures, requires considerable time until vascularization and skin grafting, is high cost, and has the possibility of infection of the graft. Nonetheless, it is an excellent option for the management of complex scalp wounds in the setting of trauma.

Tissue expansion is yet another option that can be used either alone or in tandem with skin grafting or tissue advancement flaps. The scalp is a favorable site for tissue expansion, and this may be a way in which hair-bearing areas can be preserved in lieu of scar formation that may preclude additional hair growth. The process of expansion is initiated approximately 2 weeks after insertion, and, during the expansion process, sterile saline is injected into the expander to stretch the tissues until the skin slightly blanches or until it becomes painful for the patient. The ultimate goal is to achieve an expansion circumference roughly two to three times the size of the defect, a process typically taking up to 12 weeks.

Local rotational flaps are often used in cases of large, complex scalp lacerations or wounds in the setting of trauma. The parietal scalp has the greatest amount of laxity and is a good region to incorporate into the rotational flap. A simple advancement type flap will work well for a central defect, especially in areas around the face and forehead. The flap length-to-width ratio should be less than 4:1 to prevent vascular compromise.

However, with defects involving the scalp, an advancement flap is generally not well tolerated because of the multidirectional lines of tension produced by the galea. For this reason, large, widely based rotation flaps are typically used to allow for optimal wound healing and, ultimately, good cosmetic outcomes as well. An example of a rotational flap is the O-to-Z rotation/advancement repair or, for posterior scalp defects, the V–Y advancement flap.

Finally, one of the most involved methods of scalp closure is the execution of a free flap. Some examples of muscle flaps include a latissimus dorsi and serratus anterior flaps. The latissimus dorsi is a thin, broad, well-vascularized muscle vascularized by the thoracodorsal vessels, suitable for covering a large area of cranial reconstruction. Pedicle length can be up to 10 cm, and the muscle is typically harvested without a skin paddle. Often, this free flap is covered with a skin graft. This is a nice choice for posterior scalp injuries. The serratus anterior muscle free flap can be used for smaller defects and has a vascular pedicle which can be up to 15 cm in length. Other commonly used free flaps include the radial forearm fasciocutaneous flap and the anterolateral thigh free flap. These procedures should be tailored based on patient comorbidities, defect size, distance to donor vessels, cosmesis, and feasibility with surgeon experience. A multidisciplinary approach is often required. These procedures require an extensive discussion with the patient of risks and benefits, as well as expected outcomes.

In cases where there is obvious infection and the skin defect is too large to be closed primarily, attention should be turned to wound washout and temporary wound closure with a wound VAC placed under negative pressure to assist with wound granulation and delayed reconstruction.

Pros and cons of various surgical approaches are listed in here.

- Advantages of a simple surgical closure include a shorter procedure, a quicker recovery time, it is cost- and resource-effective, and it may be appropriate for medically complex patients. Disadvantages are that if a wound is under significant tension, it may not heal and may cause more problems and require more surgeries in the future.
- The biggest advantage to a staged procedure is the ability to follow the wound closely over a long period of time and create an environment for gradual and controlled healing of the wound with the best possible cosmetic outcome. However, a patient may be too medically complex to undergo multiple surgeries or may not have the capabilities or resources to follow through with a complex surgical plan.
- A rotational muscle flap may provide a robust source of blood supply and revitalization to the overlying wound tissue. Furthermore, in the setting of a complex fracture causing a CSF leak, particularly in the posterior fossa, a muscle flap can provide a permanent solution to seal the leak off. A disadvantage of a rotational flap procedure may be surgical team inexperience and comfort level with performing such procedures, as well as cosmetic deformity/postoperative pain and limitations for the patient.

The patient we presented with the gunshot wound was managed with primary closure. Before surgery, he was positioned supine on a horseshoe headrest. This enables maximum mobility of the scalp, which is otherwise hindered by pin-fixation. The scalp was generously shaved and a bicoronal-type incision was made behind the hairline. The area of tissue destroyed by the bullet entry point was ellipsed out with a scalpel. A small craniotomy was performed to explore and repair the dural defect. The bone was replated, and the wound was copiously irrigated. The incision was closed primarily with 2-0 Vicryl and staples on the skin. Next, attention was turned to the maxillary region where the bullet was lodged. Since this was located in the superficial tissues, removal of the bullet was performed at this time, to avoid complications down the line and save the costs of a second trip to the operating room.

Oral Boards Review: Management Pearls

- With few exceptions, all full-thickness scalp wounds should be closed surgically.
- Goals of surgery include closure of the defect while preserving motor and sensory functions of the face and scalp.
- All potential options should be discussed as part of the decision-making process.
- Often, multiple surgical teams may be involved, and a planned stepwise approach may provide the best outcome for the patient.

Pivot Points

- If a patient presents with or develops local inflammatory changes, fever, and/ or neurological deficits, urgent broad-spectrum antibiotics are indicated, along with pan-cultures of blood and urine, and possibly a lumbar puncture to obtain CSF.
- If repeat imaging is warranted for clinical deterioration, careful attention should be paid to underlying bony anatomy and enhancement of the dura. In the setting of infection, venous sinus thrombosis can also occur.
- Care teams should have a low threshold for surgical re-exploration with any red flag symptoms.

Aftercare

Immediately postoperatively, there are some key pearls to optimize wound healing and patient comfort. First and foremost, a dressing such as a head wrap should typically be used (with exception in cases of free flaps) to provide full coverage of the wound and some mild pressure to reduce edema. Furthermore, elevation of the head to minimize edema is recommended. Drains are often left in place when considerable undermining of the scalp has occurred. Drains are typically left in place until output is below 30 cc/ d per drain for several days.

If the patient has had a free flap procedure, all medical staff involved in the patient's care should be educated on appropriate flap precautions. Typically, flap checks are performed every hour for at least the first postoperative day, with frequency being reduced afterward. Most free flap complications are noted to occur within the first 48 h of the procedure. The patient should be positioned so that there is no occlusive pressure applied to the flap. Furthermore, the nurses and team members should understand how and where to Doppler the flap and properly evaluate the flap for signs of flap failure (e.g., duskiness, pallor, dampened signals, etc.) and notify the surgical team immediately.

A major consideration in this patient population is also the ability to follow through with appointments beyond the inpatient setting. Much of the aftercare of complex scalp lacerations may occur on an outpatient basis. These patients may require a course of postoperative antibiotics to be continued in the outpatient setting, and there should be a clear follow-up plan regarding the duration of antibiotics. In many cases, it may be prudent to involve the infectious disease service to provide input.

It is also imperative that medically complex patients with surgically managed scalp lacerations be evaluated by an internist while in the hospital if they have comorbidities such as obesity, diabetes mellitus, arterial and venous insufficiencies (peripheral vascular disease), or are immunocompromised in any way. These are some of the greatest risk factors for poor wound healing—and it is the responsibility of the surgical team to make sure that these risk factors are addressed appropriately. Nutritional status should also be assessed, and certain patients may require supplements such as a multivitamin or vitamins A, C, and E to support wound healing.

The patient with the gunshot wound that we presented required a stay of approximately 5–7 days in a neurointensive care unit, to be managed for his acute traumatic brain injury. He was monitored closely for any evidence of CSF leak and was maintained on a course of antibiotics for several weeks given the trajectory of the bullet through the brain tissue and maxillary sinus.

Complications and Management

Prevention of complications in the management of complex scalp lacerations is key. Arguably the biggest nemesis to wound healing is infection. This can be challenging since, if infections are not recognized and dealt with promptly, bacteria can spread to the bone of the skull and cause osteomyelitis. In some cases, this may even lead to subdural empyema or full-blown meningitis. Therefore, clinicians should maintain a high suspicion for infection when a patient presents with symptoms such as new incisional pain, low-grade fevers, or wound erythema. Workup of infection should include blood work such as CBC, ESR/CRP, and blood cultures. Deeper lacerations may require additional CT and possibly subsequent MR imaging (with and without contrast) to delineate if there is evidence of infection spreading to the bone or meninges. If a patient has evidence of meningismus, lumbar puncture should be performed as well and CSF sent for cell counts and cultures. If a patient presents and meets sepsis criteria, broad-spectrum antibiotics should be started immediately. However, if surgery is planned and the patient is not actively septic, it is recommended that antibiotics be started after intraoperative cultures have been sent. Surgery should not be delayed in the setting of an infected scalp wound; however, ultimate timing is at the discretion of the attending surgeon.

Wound dehiscence and breakdown are other potential complications. There are a number of options in the surgeon's armamentarium to address such issues. A stepwise, graduated approach in terms of complexity should be used, starting with the less complex options and working toward more complex options as indicated. Please refer to the "Surgical Procedure" section for more details. Additionally, if a patient presents with an open wound that was previously surgically closed, the surgeon should attempt to identify and address the underlying issues that caused the problem to manifest.

A careful history and physical exam is imperative. For example, the patient may be in a malnourished state and may be exhibiting poor wound healing as a consequence. If there is suspicion for this, it is recommended to check nutrition labs, such as albumin and prealbumin, and obtain a nutrition evaluation consult in the hospital. Another culprit for poor wound healing may be poor hygiene or lack of compliance with the prescribed wound care regimen altogether. To prevent this, care should be taken to educate the patient on the "do's and don'ts" of scalp and wound care. Special considerations for the scalp include wearing hats and helmets, sun exposure, shampoo and hair product selections—all of which should be discussed on an individual basis. Furthermore, if it is deemed that the patient may lack the support or resources for proper care at home, every effort should be made to obtain for the patient a visiting home nurse or refer them to a rehabilitation facility for a finite period of time.

For the case we presented, hydrocephalus was a major delayed complication for which the patient was monitored. Any change in mental status prompted an immediate head CT. He was eventually discharged to rehab and otherwise had an uneventful recovery.

Oral Boards Review: Complications Pearls

- Recognizing risk factors for wound complications is key to avoiding them.
- Patient education and ensuring reliable, scheduled follow-up appointments are essential.
- The clinician should maintain a high suspicion for infection involving the central nervous system (meningitis, subdural empyema, intracranial abscess formation) in patients with complex scalp lacerations, particularly those with polytrauma.

Evidence and Outcomes

Much of the data on complex scalp laceration management are limited to clinical case series from single institutions or groups of surgeons. Nevertheless, the guiding principles of scalp reconstruction have been fairly constant over time. Keys to a successful outcome in complex scalp lacerations include clearly defining goals of surgery preoperatively and tailoring the correct operation for the patient.

Further Reading

Angelos PC, Downs BW. Options for the management of forehead and scalp defects. *Facial Plast Surg Clin N Am.* 2009 Aug;17(3):379–393.

Gurunlugolu R, Glasgow M, Arton J, Bronsert M. Retrospective analysis of facial dog bite injuries at a Level I trauma center in the Denver metro area. *J Trauma Acute Care Surg.* 2014;76(5):1294–1300.

Hamrah H, Mehrvarz S, Mirghasscmi AM. The frequency of brain CT-scan findings in patients with scalp lacerations following mild traumatic brain injury: A cross-sectional study. *Bull Emerg Trauma.* 2018 Jan;6(1):54–58.

Kruse-Losler B, Presser D, Meyer U, et al. Reconstruction of large defects on the scalp and fore-head as an interdisciplinary challenge: experience in the management of 39 cases. *Eur J Surg Oncol.* 2006;32:1006–1014.

Lee RH, Gamble WB, Robertson B, Manson PN. The MCFONTZL classification system for soft-tissue injuries to the face. *Plast Recontrc Surg.* 1999 April;103(4):1150–1157.

Occipital Condyle Fractures

Evan Fitchett, Fadi Alsaiegh, and Jack Jallo

21

Case Presentation

A 38-year-old woman presents to the emergency department (ED) via ambulance after a motor vehicle accident (MVA). She was a restrained driver and collided with a parked vehicle at roughly 30 mph. EMS reported loss of consciousness at the scene, but on presentation she is awake, alert, and oriented to person, place, and time. In the ED, she complains of diffuse neck and back pain that is slightly worse in her high cervical spine. Initial trauma workup is only significant for airbag chemical burns on her face and a small abrasion on her left forehead. She has no medical conditions, nor does she have a preexisting spine deformity or known osseous defects. Initial x-rays of the head, neck, and spine are negative for any injury, but CT of head and cervical spine shows a small, linear, nondisplaced fracture at the right occipital condyle with minimal extension into the occiput.

Questions

1. Which imaging modalities are most sensitive in detecting occipital condyle fractures (OCF)?
2. What follow-up imaging is required and why?
3. What are the classifications of occipital condyle fractures?

Assessment and Planning

Neck and back pain in the setting of an acute traumatic event includes a significant differential diagnosis, such as ligamentous injury; any number of bone fractures, including OCF; and muscle strains. The range in severity is broad, and the most consequential sequela involve injury to the spinal cord or exiting nerves.

OCF continue to be a rather uncommon occurrence, found in as low as 0.4% to as high as 16% of traumas. When OCF do occur, they are typically in the setting of a blunt trauma, as in an MVA, or through significant axial loading, as in a diving accident. Thin slice CT scan evaluating the head and neck is now routine in trauma centers, but special consideration should be made to evaluate for this rare type of fracture because it can be easily missed on plain films or lower resolution CT images. When OCF is discovered on initial CT scan, the craniocervical junction should be stabilized with an external rigid collar until further evaluation is carried out. There are two major considerations when assessing the need for surgical intervention. First is evidence of neurological injury, particularly damage to the lower cranial nerves or evidence of brainstem compression at the level of the foramen magnum. Second, it is important to classify the fracture as stable or unstable with respect to the craniocervical junction. This requires thorough evaluation of the CT scan with reconstructions looking for bilateral OCF, evidence of atlanto-occipital distraction, and then follow-up MRI to evaluate the integrity of the craniocervical ligaments. Special attention should be paid to those fractures with avulsed fragments, particularly those displaced medially, which may be pressing on the spinal cord and brainstem. The vast majority of patients will have a stable craniocervical junction in the setting of OCF and can be treated conservatively. If there are any signs of ligamentous injury and/or instability, then management requires more invasive options. Because OCF occur most commonly in the setting of trauma, thorough imaging of the rest of the spine and possibly even vascular imaging of vertebral arteries is indicated to assess for concomitant injury.

Oral Boards Review: Diagnostic Pearls

- Signs and symptoms of an OCF are often nonspecific, and elevated suspicion in traumatic injury, particularly high-speed impacts such as in MVAs, should prompt careful evaluation of the occiput on CT scan. Classification of fracture type can be documented, but current evidence suggests that apart from avulsed/displaced type fractures, these classifications may play a smaller role in surgical decision making than previously thought. There are two commonly used classification systems, one by Tuli and another by Anderson and Montesano.
    - Tuli:
        - Type 1: A nondisplaced fracture that is most often considered stable. Displacement is measured as a distance of less than 2 mm.
        - Type 2A: Displaced fracture without ligamentous injury or evidence of instability.
        - Type 2B: Displaced fracture with ligamentous injury and evidence of craniocervical instability.
    - Anderson and Montesano:
        - Type 1: Impacted fracture, commonly the result of axial loading from MVA or diving accidents. Special attention should be paid to the integrity of the contralateral alar ligament.
        - Type 2: Basilar occipital fracture that extends through the occipital condyle. Again, alar ligament integrity should be evaluated as disruption of this ligament leads to craniocervical instability. The extension of the fracture into other portions of the occiput can put cranial nerves exiting nearby foramina at increased risk of injury.
        - Type 3: Avulsion fracture from extreme rotation and/or lateral bending. There is often instability in this type of fracture as it typically results in disruption of the alar ligament (Figure 21.1).
- If an OCF is present, it is important to assess for lower cranial nerve deficits, particularly damage to the hypoglossal nerve, but also cranial nerves IX, X,

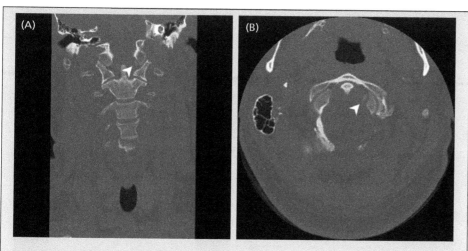

Figure 21.1 Coronal (A) and axial (B) sections of a cervical spine CT scan demonstrating a Type III left occipital condyle fracture with a medially displaced, avulsed bone fragment (*white arrow*).

and XI as they exit at the jugular foramen near the occipital condyles. These deficits can be present on admission or develop days to weeks later.
- Though CT scan of the craniocervical elements provides the fastest and most sensitive imaging modality for diagnosis of OCF, MRI of the craniocervical junction is important to assess for ligamentous injury that could contribute to instability.
- Due to the mechanism of injury, OCF often occur concomitantly with other injuries, such as central cord syndrome and fractures of vertebral elements at lower levels.

Questions

1. What are the clinical indications for surgical intervention in these patients?
2. How does concomitant injury to other portions of the cervical spine contribute to surgical decision making?

Decision Making

While most patients with OCF will not require surgical intervention, it is important to know when invasive methods of fracture stabilization are warranted. Immediate causes of concern include displaced or avulsed fractures (i.e., Anderson and Montesano type 3 fracture, particularly those directed medially toward the brainstem); bilateral OCF; ligamentous injury with signs of instability such as occiput–C1 distraction; or focal neurological deficits in a cranial nerve. Misalignment can be evaluated on CT by measuring a distance between the condyle and atlas of greater than 2 mm. Instability can be evaluated by observing mobility of the atlantooccipital joint on flexion and extension imaging or evidence of alar ligament injury on MRI.

When one of the previous indications of instability is noted, the next decision is regarding internal versus external fixation with a Halo device. Both have good outcomes for pain control and stabilization of the cranicervical junction, preventing progression or onset of delayed neurological deficits. If obvious neural compression is present, then surgical decompression is warranted. There is limited data comparing Halo to internal fixation for these patients, nor is there good evidence to suggest to which level internal fixation should extend, though occiput to C2 or C3 is typical.

Questions

1. In the setting of internal fixation and stabilization of the craniocervical joint, should instrumentation be permanent or temporary until the joint is stabilized?
2. How does concomitant injury to other parts of the vertebral column modify surgical planning?

Surgical Procedure

Escalation of management to surgical intervention should only be considered in the setting of atlanto-occipital ligamentous injury or craniocervical instability. The vast majority of patients will not have either of these elements and will benefit from conservative management with external cervical immobilization. When surgical intervention is indicated, either Halo-vest immobilization or internal fixation of the craniocervical junction can be offered.

Internal fixation is performed with patients placed in the prone position with head fixation in Mayfield pins. The head should be in midline, with slight flexion to permit easy dissection and adequate access to the vertebral elements from the occiput to the lower cervical vertebrae. Repositioning under fluoroscopic guidance for final fixation can be used to optimize surgical results. Monitoring of somatosensory evoked potentials (SSEPs) and motor evoked potentials (MEPs) is recommended. Exposure should be performed with care to minimize disruption of the intrinsic muscles of the neck and occiput. Fixation alone or fixation with decompression of neural elements is usually performed from the occiput to C2 or C3. The length of the construct depends on the extent of injury. The goal is to achieve stability with the shortest construct possible in order to preserve as much mobility as possible. As for any internal fixation procedure, it is important to carefully evaluate the bony anatomy, including the thickness of the occiput to avoid any cerebellar or vascular injury.

Oral Boards Review: Management Pearls

- Premature discontinuation of rigid collar or Halo immobilization can result in cranial nerve deficits, nystagmus, diplopia, vertigo, and other symptoms. These deficits can resolve or improve after resumption of immobilization in a timely fashion.

- Nonoperative treatment with external immobilization is almost always sufficient to achieve bony fusion and recovery of cranial nerve deficits.
- Surgical instrumentation should be strongly considered in those with bilateral OCF.

Pivot Points

- The management guidelines set forth by the AHRQ recommend external immobilization with at least a rigid collar for all OCF. If bilateral OCF is present, then more rigid immobilization may be indicated with a Halo vest or similar device.
- If there is evidence of ligamentous injury resulting in craniocervical instability, then either Halo or surgical options, such as internal fixation, are appropriate.
- If there is concomitant injury to other portions of the cervical bony elements, extension of the instrumentation to these levels may be warranted.

Aftercare

The follow-up care of patients suffering from OCF varies widely depending on the modality of management initially performed. Most patients will progress well with conservative management when indicated. Follow-up care for these patients requires a thorough neurological exam because cranial nerve deficits can develop days to weeks later. There remains debate on the length of time required for external immobilization with either a rigid collar or Halo device. As little as 6 weeks in a rigid collar or 3 months in a Halo device appear to provide enough time for stabilization and recovery from the fracture. Most surgeons will use radiographic follow-up to guide their decision regarding the length of immobilization. In surgically managed patients, there also continues to be debate regarding the permanency of fixation. For patients with osteoporosis or poor bone quality, autologous bone graft (e.g., hip graft) can be used. Additionally, the use of bone stimulators can be considered.

Complications and Management

As with any surgical interventions, postoperative complications such as infection, urinary retention, and damage to the intrinsic muscles of the neck and occiput can occur. Urinary retention is usually self-limited, and there should be little concern for significant neurological injury in the setting of isolated urinary retention with no other neurological deficits. As with any surgical intervention, particularly with instrumentation, there is a risk of infection. The most concerning complications are continued or new-onset lower cranial nerve palsy, spinal cord injury in the setting of evolving signs of myelopathy, and vertebral artery injury.

Oral Boards Review: Complication Pearls

1. The most concerning complication of OCF is injury to the brainstem or lower cranial nerves. Nervous system injury can be transient or permanent and can appear days to weeks after initial injury.

Evidence and Outcomes

There continues to be limited prospective analysis of treatment options for OCF, and much of the data are limited to small case series or retrospective analysis. Some larger retrospective studies have attempted to contribute long-term follow-up data to the literature by analyzing how various fracture types were treated and their outcomes. The evidence continues to suggest that external immobilization with a rigid collar is a safe and effective treatment modality for patients without evidence of craniocervical instability or misalignment and in patients without neurological sequela or bilateral OCF. Whereas internal surgical fixation should be reserved for patients with displaced fractures, other significant injury to the atlanto-axial-occipital joint and/or cervical spine, or evidence of craniocervical instability and misalignment. Overall, patients qualifying for conservative management with external fixation tend to perform well at follow-up with minimal residual pain.

Further Reading

Bystrom O, Jensen T, Poulsen F. Outcome of conservatively treated occipital condylar fractures: A retrospective study. *J Craniovertebr Junction Spine*. 2017;8(4): 322–327. doi: 10.4103/jcvjs. jcvjs_97_17. https://www.ncbi.nlm.nih.gov/pmc/articles/PMC5763588/

Clayman D, Sykes C, Vines F. Occipital condyle fractures: Clinical presentation and radiological detection. 1994. *Am Soc Neuroradiol*. 1994;15:1309–1315. https://pdfs.semanticscholar.org/37e8/857e7d3e917cc816ffd3c1daf3c4d6a599c7.pdf

Kruger A, Oberkircher L, Frangen T, Ruchholtz S, Kuhne C, Junge A. Fractures of the occipital condyle: Clinical spectrum and course in eight patients. *J Craniovertebr Junction Spine*. 2013;4(2):49–55. doi: 10.4103/0974-8237.128525. https://www.ncbi.nlm.nih.gov/pmc/articles/PMC3980555/

Maserati MB, Stephens B, Zohny Z, et al. Occipital condyle fractures: Clinical decision rule and surgical management. *J Neurosurg Spine*. 2009 Oct;11(4):388–95. doi: 10.3171/2009.5.SPINE08866. https://www.ncbi.nlm.nih.gov/pubmed/19929333

Rumboldt Z, Cianfoni A, Varma A. *Clinical Imaging of Spinal Trauma: A Case-Based Approach*. New York: Cambridge University Press, 2018: 38–39.

Theodore N, Arabi B, Dhall Sanjay, et al. Occipital condyle fractures. *Neurosurgery*. 2013;72:106–113. doi: 10.1227/neu.0b013e3182775527. https://www.ncbi.nlm.nih.gov/pubmed/?term=10.1227%2Fneu.0b013e3182775527

Waseem M, Upadhyay R, Al-Husayne H, Agyare S. Occipital condyle fracture in a patient with neck pain. *Int J Emerg Med*. 2014;7:5. doi: 10.1186/1865-1280-7-5. https://www.ncbi.nlm.nih.gov/pmc/articles/PMC3899382/

Multimodality Monitoring in Severe Traumatic Brain Injury

Abdelhakim Khellaf, Peter J. A. Hutchinson, and Adel Helmy

22

Case Presentation

A 20-year-old, right-handed woman presented to the emergency department following a road traffic accident. The patient was a pedestrian who was struck at night by a bus traveling at 40 mph. Medical first responders noted a Glasgow Coma Scale (GCS) score of 7 on scene (E1, V1, M5) and pupils were 3 mm bilaterally and reactive to light. The patient was intubated and ventilated upon transfer to a local hospital and is emergently brought to the nearest major trauma center (MTC). On arrival to the MTC, the patient was managed according to the Advanced Trauma and Life Support (ATLS) protocol. She was adequately ventilated and hemodynamically stable (heart rate 81 and blood pressure 110/75 mm Hg), but remained comatose (GCS 7) with no change in pupillary function. External examination revealed ecchymosis around the mastoid process bilaterally and extensive bruising over the scalp, left shoulder, and abdomen. Toxin screening and β-hCG were negative.

Questions

1. What is the most appropriate imaging modality in this context?
2. What are the most appropriate anatomical areas to image, and why?
3. What is the most likely diagnosis?
4. Which vascular structures might be at risk of injury?

Traumatic brain injury (TBI) is a major determinant of morbidity and mortality; it is the commonest cause of death in people younger than 40 years of age in developed countries and the cause of death in half of major trauma patients. In the context of trauma, CT is the fundamental clinical modality due to its easy availability, sensitivity to hemorrhage, ability to assess the cervical spine, and the ability to assess body trauma at the same time.

Angiography may be appropriate in some circumstances, including skull base fracture traversing the carotid canal; C-spine fracture encroaching on transverse foramina of C2–C6, where the vertebral artery runs; penetrating head or neck injury; and clinical suspicion of vascular injury (e.g., acute Horner syndrome).

CT angiography is a sensitive screening test; however, formal digital subtraction angiography (DSA) is the gold standard. MRI can provide much more detailed information

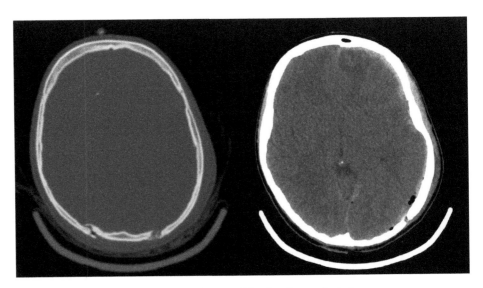

Figure 22.1 Noncontrast enhanced CT of the head on admission.

about axonal injury, microhemorrhages at the gray–white matter junction indicative of diffuse brain injury, and brainstem injury, all of which are poorly visualized by CT. Access to MRI is logistically difficult in the acutely unstable patient and much more limited than access to CT.[1]

In this case, a noncontrast CT scan of the head (Figure 22.1) was performed per ATLS guidelines. It revealed the features shown in Figure 22.1:

- Left-sided thin acute subdural hematoma (ASDH) with 5 mm midline shift
- Bifrontal contusion
- Comminuted depressed fracture of lambdoid suture bilaterally extending into left occipital and left petrous part of the temporal bone, with the fracture line reaching to the carotid canal as well as the left transverse sinus (TS)/sigmoid sinus (SS) junction. There was no sphenoid or ethmoid bone involvement.

Key points on skull base fractures are presented in the following pearls.[1–5]

Oral Boards Review: Diagnosis Pearls

- Base of the skull fractures typically suggest significant forces sustained by the cranium and can present with periorbital ecchymosis ("raccoon eyes"), ecchymosis around the mastoid process ("Battle's sign"), rhinorrhea, and/or otorrhea.
- In cases of fractures involving the petrous bone, high suspicion for vascular injury to the petrous segment (C2) of the internal carotid artery (ICA) warrants prompt vascular imaging (usually CT angiography due to accessibility and accuracy); relatedly, fractures involving the foramen spinosum might lead to laceration of the middle meningeal artery.
- In the eventuality of bleeding of the C2 segment of the ICA intraoperatively with no previous scan, packing the area tightly might be one of the only

---

options to allow sufficient time to perform an emergent cerebral angiogram with endovascular control, like stenting.

- Administration of a polyvalent pneumococcal vaccine (e.g., the 23-valent Pneumovax) as prophylactic treatment for posttraumatic meningitis is indicated in patients suffering of traumatic skull base fractures due to risk of CSF leak.

In our case example patient, the CT scan of the spine does not reveal any abnormality. Additional important findings from the CT trauma survey (chest, abdomen, and pelvis) show a left grade 1 kidney laceration, a subtle mesenteric contusion at the left iliac fossa with no active abdominal bleeding, and a left closed proximal humeral fracture requiring fixation. Management of a severely injured major trauma patient involves concurrent care with multiple other services (in this case, general surgery and orthopedic surgery). Thus, effective communication and clinical prioritization depending on severity are crucial.

Questions

1. What are the main components of brain multimodality monitoring (MMM) in severe TBI (sTBI), and what can they measure?
2. What are your clinical targets for:
    a. Mean intracranial pressure (ICP)?
    b. Cerebral perfusion pressure (CPP)?
    c. Brain tissue oxygen tension?
    d. Brain lactate/pyruvate ratio?
3. What is pressure reactivity index (PRx), and what is its clinical relevance?

Assessment and Planning

The patient was put under general anaesthesia and neuromuscular blockade and immediately transferred from the neurocritical care unit (NCCU) to the neurosurgical theater for ICP bolt insertion. The patient received prophylactic IV antibiotics and was appropriately prepped and draped. The neurosurgeon opted for a right frontal approach (due to preference for the nondominant hemisphere, noneloquent brain) and performed a twist drill burr hole with brace anteriorly to the coronal suture. The access device allows transmission of an ICP monitor (Codman), a brain tissue oxygenation probe (Licox), and a cerebral microdialysis (CMD) catheter into the brain parenchyma; all catheters were secured. The measured opening pressure was 13 mm Hg. The patient was then returned to the NCCU for further care.

The central tenets of closed TBI management are control of ICP and maintenance of adequate delivery of glucose and oxygen to the brain, which are achieved through effective neurocritical care. Using multiple brain monitors, a method termed *brain multimodality monitoring*, can provide individualized refinement of therapeutic targets and identify specific pathological derangements in patients. Brain MMM in patients with sTBI is an important tool that helps to optimize conditions for brain recovery and prevent secondary injury. Considerations during clinical interpretation of brain MMM include the following. (1) Focal monitors may not be representative of the whole brain given their placement in a specific locality. Knowledge of the probes' location and the patient's clinical context is critical in interpreting multimodality data. (2) Care must be taken in interpreting data from areas adjacent to a focal mass lesion. Cross-sectional imaging to determine the location of monitors is helpful in interpretation.

In our center, we aim to provide all patients with sTBI intracranial MMM within 4 h of admission to the NCCU, if patients are suitably stable, as standard of care. A dedicated interface software is used for data acquisition and processing of multimodality neuromonitoring inputs. We currently have extensive experience with the Intensive Care Monitoring+ (ICM+) software developed by the Brain Physics laboratory at the University of Cambridge. It provides real-time neuromonitoring trends and multiple, derived neurophysiology indices (e.g., PRx) for clinical applications at the bedside and for retrospective analysis.[6] (See Figure 22.2 for a typical example of ICM+ output.) Similar software is commercially available, such as CNS Monitor and BedmasterEx.[7,8]

ICP Monitoring

The Monro-Kellie doctrine states that the sum of volumes of brain, CSF, and intracranial blood content should remain fixed within a rigid cranium; as such, increase in one of these components should result in a decrease/displacement in the remaining two.[9] ICP monitoring, which can help identify growth of mass lesions or worsening brain swelling, is a cornerstone in the evaluation of the patient with sTBI who is often paralyzed and sedated and in whom clinical evaluation is limited.

The most recent Brain Trauma Foundation (BTF) guidelines for the management of sTBI (4th Edition, September 2016), endorsed by the American Association of Neurological Surgeons and the Congress of Neurological Surgeons, thoroughly evaluated available evidence and translated it into practical recommendations.

The BTF guidelines suggest invasive ICP monitoring in all "salvageable" TBI patients presenting with a GCS 8 or less and an abnormal CT scan (Level IIB recommendation) to "reduce in-hospital and 2-week post-injury mortality" (Level IIB). ICP monitoring is also indicated in sTBI patients with a normal CT scan if two or more of the following are noted at admission: age older than 40 years, unilateral or bilateral motor posturing, and systolic blood pressure of less than 90 mm Hg.[10] In our unit, we routinely utilize invasive ICP monitoring in all patients with sTBI who are clinically salvageable and cannot be clinically monitored (e.g., multiply injured patients requiring sedation).

Invasive ICP monitoring is the gold standard because noninvasive ICP monitoring methods, such as ultrasound evaluation of the optic nerve sheath diameter (ONSD), do not provide the same degree of accuracy and continuity. ICP can be invasively monitored in a variety of locations including the subarachnoid, subdural, or epidural space. While intraventricular probes are considered the gold standard because they are less likely to demonstrate gradients between the intracranial compartments, intraparenchymal monitoring is more easily delivered and is utilized in our unit. An external ventricular drain (EVD) allows for both global measurement of ICP and treatment of elevated ICP via CSF drainage, but these benefits are mitigated by the risks of misplacement, infection, and hemorrhage. An intraparenchymal probe allows good accuracy (although less than

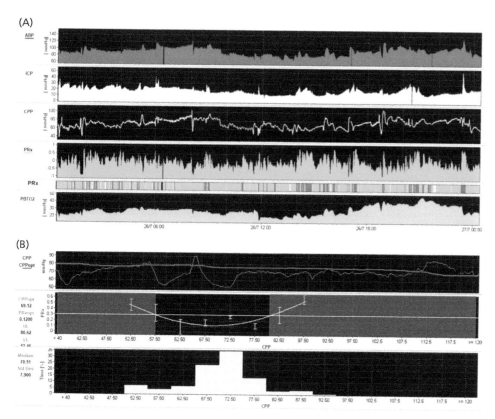

Figure 22.2 (A) A 24-h direct output from ICM+ software with plotting of ABP, intracranial pressure (ICP), cerebral perfusion pressure (CPP), pressure reactivity index (PRx; moving correlation coefficient between ABP and ICP), and brain tissue oxygenation (PbtO$_2$), respectively, from top to bottom.

(B) A 3-h direct output from ICM+ software with CPP$_{opt}$ algorithm in the case described.

Top: Plotting of real CPP trend against calculated CPP$_{opt}$ trend over time.
Middle: Plotting of mean PRx against CPP; Calculated CPP$_{opt}$ represents the CPP value at which PRx is minimized according to a pre-established algorithm (i.e., CPP value at which cerebral autoregulation is thought to be best preserved).
Bottom: Percentage of 3-h period the patient has spent at each CPP 5 mm Hg bin.

With thanks to Dr. Erta Beqiri and Dr. Peter Smielewski for providing these images.

an intraventricular probe) and the possibility to integrate other brain monitors during bolt placement—but no CSF drainage. Of note, coagulopathy remains a relative contra-indication to invasive ICP monitoring and may lead to a short delay while hematological parameters are corrected.

We generally use mean ICP as our main goal-directed measure. Pathologic ICP thresholds are reported as between greater than 20 and 25 mm Hg across studies. The current consensus among experts is to keep ICP below 20 mm Hg. The BTF characterizes the mean ICP therapeutic threshold which should be treated at more than 22 mm Hg (Level IIB recommendation from mostly observational evidence, no Level I) as values above it are associated with increased mortality.[10]

The landmark Trial of Intracranial-Pressure Monitoring in Traumatic Brain Injury, by Chesnut et al. (2012) is the only randomized controlled trial in sTBI patients evaluating outcomes of ICP monitoring–driven therapy versus management without ICP monitoring (using imaging/clinical examination). The trial failed to show an overall significant difference in outcomes between the two groups, although the study has received a great deal of criticism. Outcomes were defined by a 21-component weighted composite score with 12/21 included tests of primarily neuropsychologic nature. Moreover, the study showed nonsignificant benefits in survival and functional outcomes tested with the extended Glasgow Outcome Scale (GOS-E) favoring the ICP monitoring group.[11] This trial suffered from important drawbacks, including study conduct in countries with limited prehospital care (Bolivia and Ecuador) and limited experience of neurological monitoring, with a high risk of type II error. Furthermore, ICP was treated in both groups and this was not, therefore, a study of whether ICP should be treated in patients with moderate to severe TBI. Nonetheless, it remains to this day the only major attempt to produce Class 1 evidence for ICP-driven management—considering the pivotal role of ICP monitoring in severe TBI.[10,12]

Interpretation of ICP changes in an individual patient goes further than looking at a mean trend.

ICP waveform can add additional valuable information on the pathologic changes occurring in intracranial hypertension and should be considered whenever possible.

Central Perfusion Pressure Monitoring and Pressure Reactivity Index

Recall the key equation CPP = MAP − ICP, where MAP is *mean arterial pressure*.

CPP constitutes the pressure gradient across the cerebral vascular system. It can be derived using ICP monitoring and invasive arterial monitoring. BTF guidelines recommend CPP monitoring to guide therapy in sTBI patients (Level IIB recommendation); the suggested CPP target is 60–70 mm Hg (Level IIB recommendation). Of note, increased CPP (>70 mm Hg) after sTBI has been associated with a higher risk of acute respiratory distress syndrome (ARDS).[10]

Cerebral autoregulation is the capacity to maintain cerebral blood flow over a wide range of CPP through homeostatic vascular changes. If cerebrovascular autoregulation is intact, the vascular tree can regulate the vascular supply based on tissue demand. In case of an increase in MAP, vasoconstriction of the cerebral vasculature maintains constant cerebral blood flow. Consequently, vasoconstriction reduces the arterial blood volume and should decrease ICP. However, this autoregulation relationship between ICP and MAP is disturbed in TBI, where increases in MAP can lead to increases in ICP.[13,14]

The PRx provides an ICP-derived metric of cerebrovascular autoregulation; it is a moving correlation coefficient between ICP and MAP. PRx values typically range from −1 to 1; values above 0.25 are suggestive of impaired cerebrovascular autoregulation.[14]

CPP_{opt} represents an optimal CPP value at which autoregulation is best preserved, a concept introduced by Steiner et al. in 2002.[15] Using PRx as a surrogate for cerebrovascular autoregulation, CPP_{opt} is the evolving CPP value which minimizes PRx over a given period of time (see Figure 22.2B), and different algorithms have been described to calculate CPP_{opt}.

The CPP_{opt} Guided Therapy Assessment of Target Effectiveness (COGiTATE) study is an ongoing multicenter, phase II nonblinded, randomized controlled trial. It aims to assess the safety and feasibility of maintaining CPP at an individualized target (CPP_{opt} obtained via an automated algorithm slightly modified from Liu et al., 2017[16]) as opposed to the "one-size-fits-all" concept proposed by the current BTF guidelines (target of 60–70 mm Hg) in sTBI patients requiring ICP monitoring.[17] This will provide important insight on the feasibility of the individualized autoregulation-oriented therapy concept in sTBI patients.[14,16,18]

Brain Tissue Oxygenation Monitoring

Brain hypoxia is a major independent predictor of poor outcome. We use low brain tissue oxygen tension (i.e., partial pressure of oxygen in the cerebral tissue: $PbtO_2$) as an indicator of hypoxia. A brain tissue oxygenation probe, first described using an electrode by Clark et al. in the 1950s, is used to measure $PbtO_2$. Common commercially available probes include LICOX (Integra LifeSciences)[19] and Raumedic Neurovent-PTO[20] probes, usually placed within the brain parenchyma. By consensus, the $PbtO_2$ threshold used to indicate hypoxia is less than 20 mm Hg.

Recall that the main variables influencing blood oxygen content are primarily the fraction of inspired oxygen (FiO_2) and hemoglobin. Locally, the main factors influencing $PbtO_2$ are oxygen delivery to brain tissue, oxygen diffusion within tissue, and oxygen consumption by tissue.

The Brain Tissue Oxygen Monitoring and Management in Severe Traumatic Brain Injury-Phase 2 (BOOST-II) trial by Okonkwo et al., published in 2017, demonstrated feasibility and nonfutility of $PbtO_2$-targeted management + ICP-driven therapy when compared to ICP-driven therapy alone. A significant reduction in hypoxia burden (74%) during hospitalization in the $PbtO_2$-informed treatment group was reported with no safety issues.

When critical thresholds of ICP (>20 mm Hg for >5 min) and/or $PbtO_2$ (< 20 mm Hg for >5 min) were attained, directed interventions were used for either ICP control, $PbtO_2$ control, or both depending on the study group. ICP control, which was overall similar in both groups, comprised a wide range of measures, including adjustments to head of bed, targeted increase in CPP, therapeutic hypothermia, hypertonic saline, $PaCO_2$ targeting through adjustments in ventilation, and, rarely, last-tier therapies such as pentobarbital coma and decompressive craniectomy (DC).[21]

The third phase of the randomized study (BOOST-3) is approved and preparing for enrollment across 45 sites in the United States. It will evaluate the clinical efficacy of "a treatment protocol based on PbtO2 monitoring compared to treatment based on ICP monitoring alone."[22]

Cerebral Microdialysis

CMD allows direct measure of extracellular metabolic substrates through a semi-permeable–ended intraparenchymal catheter. MDialysis (from Sweden) provides the only approved microdialysis machine, the ISCUSflex. A microdialysis pump provides standardized perfusion fluid to the catheter. Subsequently, extracellular fluid is collected into a microvial which is usually changed every hour and sent for analysis in the ISCUSflex (refer to Figure 22.3). ISCUSflex can provide measurement of six analytes (glucose, glutamate, glycerol, lactate, pyruvate, lactate-to-pyruvate ratio) to profile trends in the patient's brain biochemistry.[23]

The brain lactate-to-pyruvate ratio (commonly, the LP ratio or LPR) is a measure of the cellular redox state (i.e., reduction–oxidation equilibrium). It reflects the balance

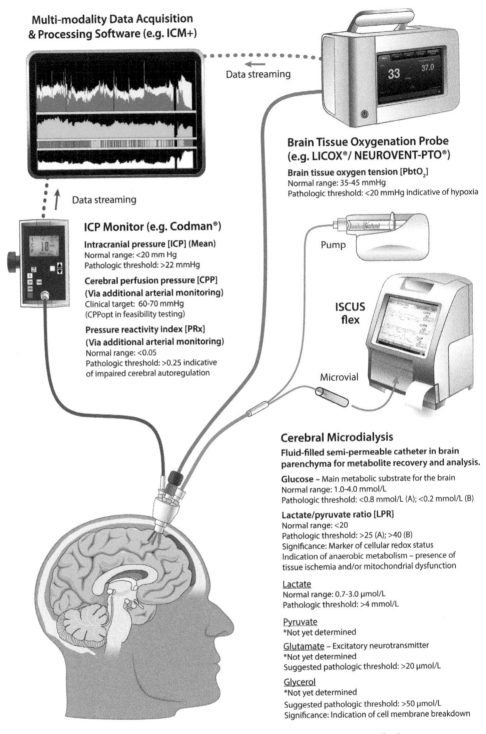

Multi-modality Data Acquisition & Processing Software (e.g. ICM+)

Data streaming

Data streaming

ICP Monitor (e.g. Codman®)

Intracranial pressure [ICP] (Mean)
Normal range: <20 mm Hg
Pathologic threshold: >22 mmHg

Cerebral perfusion pressure [CPP]
(Via additional arterial monitoring)
Clinical target: 60-70 mmHg
(CPPopt in feasibility testing)

Pressure reactivity index [PRx]
(Via additional arterial monitoring)
Normal range: <0.05
Pathologic threshold: >0.25 indicative
of impaired cerebral autoregulation

Brain Tissue Oxygenation Probe
(e.g. LICOX®/ NEUROVENT-PTO®)

Brain tissue oxygen tension [PbtO₂]
Normal range: 35-45 mmHg
Pathologic threshold: <20 mmHg indicative of hypoxia

Pump

**ISCUS
flex**

Microvial

Cerebral Microdialysis

Fluid-filled semi-permeable catheter in brain
parenchyma for metabolite recovery and analysis.

Glucose – Main metabolic substrate for the brain
Normal range: 1.0-4.0 mmol/L
Pathologic threshold: <0.8 mmol/L (A); <0.2 mmol/L (B)

Lactate/pyruvate ratio [LPR]
Normal range: <20
Pathologic threshold: >25 (A); >40 (B)
Significance: Marker of cellular redox status
Indication of anaerobic metabolism – presence of
tissue ischemia and/or mitochondrial dysfunction

Lactate
Normal range: 0.7-3.0 μmol/L
Pathologic threshold: >4 mmol/L

Pyruvate
*Not yet determined

Glutamate – Excitatory neurotransmitter
*Not yet determined
Suggested pathologic threshold: >20 μmol/L

Glycerol
*Not yet determined
Suggested pathologic threshold: >50 μmol/L
Significance: Indication of cell membrane breakdown

Figure 22.3 "Looking through a black box." A practical overview of select intraparenchymal cerebral monitors in severe traumatic brain injury.

With thanks to Mr. Philip Ball for his collaboration on this figure.

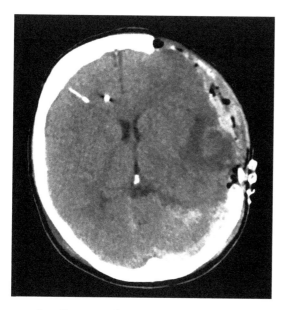

Figure 22.4 Postoperative CT scan of the head with a right frontal intraparenchymal probe in situ.

between aerobic and anaerobic metabolisms occurring locally in the brain. An LP ratio of greater than 25 is suggestive of tissue ischemia, and an LP ratio of less than 25 has been shown to correlate with good functional outcomes.[24,25] The Consensus statement from the 2014 International Microdialysis Forum suggested a tiered approach to CMD analytes: "Glucose and LP ratio [are] more clinically useful than glutamate and glycerol in TBI and SAH patients."[25] Figure 22.3 presents the target values and clinical significance of routinely used CMD analytes (from the 2014 International Microdialysis Forum)[25] within the context of MMM.

Further large multicenter prospective studies with a multimodal approach are warranted to better profile normal and pathologic values of CMD analytes and to evaluate associations with patient and tissue outcomes.

In the case described, the ICP treatment protocol for TBI patients was started, with instructions to wean sedation if ICP remained stable.

If ICP remains stable, the patient can proceed with a planned interval CT head to assess the progression of contusions in 48 h. If any acute increases in ICP are identified, a repeat CT head with CT angiogram (CTA) and CT venogram (CTV) to image the cerebral vasculature would be required. A stepwise approach to escalation/de-escalation in the management of raised ICP was carefully employed.

Oral Boards Review: Management Pearls

Is hypothermia after TBI truly beneficial?

- The large multicenter RCT Eurotherm3235 on hypothermia for patients with intracranial hypertension after TBI, published in 2015, showed that therapeutic moderate hypothermia (32–35°C) plus standard care to reduce ICP did result in slightly increased mortality outcomes compared to those with standard care alone.

- A Cochrane Review on mild hypothermia in severe brain injury, which included 37 studies with 3,110 participants (current to March 2016), demonstrated no high-quality evidence that hypothermia reduces mortality and morbidity in patients with TBI.

- The multicenter Prophylactic Hypothermia Trial to Lessen Traumatic Brain Injury–Randomized Clinical Trial (POLAR-RCT), published in October 2018, was designed to determine outcomes of early, prophylactic, sustained hypothermia (33–35°C) for at least 72 h and up to 7 days in patients with sTBI. The intent-to-treat population included a total of 500 patients (baseline) with sTBI randomized to either early hypothermia ($n = 260$) or normothermia ($n = 240$). It demonstrated no benefits from early prophylactic hypothermia in neurological outcomes and mortality at 6 months when compared to normothermia. Further, as per intent-to-treat analysis, rates of pneumonia were significantly higher in the hypothermia group (55.0%) than in the normothermia group (51.3%).

- The most recent BTF guidelines on the management of sTBI underline a significant disparity between hypothermia interventions across higher quality studies. Thus, only a Level IIB recommendation (no Level I) is included: "Early (within 2.5 hours), short-term (48 hours post-injury) prophylactic hypothermia is not recommended to improve outcomes in patients with diffuse injury."

- At our center, given limited evidence, the current practice is to restrict therapeutic hypothermia to selected patients with intracranial hypertension refractory to sedation, paralysis, and moderate hyperventilation, with close monitoring. (The key articles on hypothermia after severe TBI are reviewed by the Brain Trauma Foundation,[10] Andrews et al.,[26] Lewis et al.,[27] and Cooper et al.[28])

The following day, ICP was noted to be persistently above 20 mm Hg and not responding to sedation boluses. The LP ratio remained above 25 with occasional spikes throughout the day, indicating impaired metabolism. A 5% saline IV bolus at 2 mL/kg was attempted with limited response for a few minutes before re-increase. The P_{CO_2} level was kept at 4.39 kPa. Propofol infusion at 18 mL/h and fentanyl infusion at 7 mL/h were ongoing. The patient was normothermic, with a temperature of 36.5 °C.

At that time, a decision was made to escalate the protocol and to start 5% IV saline at 2 mL/kg (until plasma sodium >160 mmol/L or plasma osmolality ~320 mOsm/kg) along with an atracurium infusion. Atracurium is an intermediate-duration nondepolarizing neuromuscular blocking agent (NBMA) with no active metabolites, commonly used as paralytic. Hypotension and tachycardia from plasma histamine release are its main potential side effects.[29,30] No attempt to institute therapeutic hypothermia was made at this stage.

On day 2 post-injury, the patient remained paralyzed and sedated with burst suppression on bispectral index (BIS). Serum sodium level was kept at 160 mmol/

L. The protocol was further escalated and antiepileptic levetiracetam commenced in case the patient's intracranial hypertension was related to unrecognized post-traumatic seizures.

Decision Making

In this case, ICP transiently responded to hyperventilation but remained high at 30 mm Hg and was refractory to all available medical management options. Coagulation studies revealed a prothrombin time at 14.8. Given the worsening ICP refractory to maximal medical therapy, the neurosurgeon considered a DC as the next step. A DC is a surgical intervention in which a portion of the skull is removed and the dura opened (durotomy). A unilateral hemicraniectomy is generally preferred in case of a clear mass lesion; a bifrontal craniectomy can be performed in the context of diffuse injury.[31,32] After discussion with the patient's family and the neurocritical care team, informed consent to surgery was obtained from the next of kin.

Key Studies on DC

The multicenter, prospective, randomized Trial of Decompressive Craniectomy for Traumatic Intracranial Hypertension (RESCUEicp) by Hutchinson et al. (2016) examined the effectiveness of DC (bifrontal or large unilateral) versus medical therapy (including barbiturate coma) as a last-tier therapy for patients with severe, sustained, and refractory posttraumatic intracranial hypertension. This study showed that DC for patients with this condition resulted in significant benefits in mortality at both 6 and 12 months, but higher rates of vegetative state and more severe lower and upper disability on GOS-E compared to medical management.[31] Results of this study were released after completion of the most recent BTF Guidelines. Recruitment for another multicenter randomized controlled trial, the Randomised Evaluation of Surgery with Craniectomy for patients Undergoing Evacuation of Acute SubDural Haematoma (RESCUE-ASDH), is still ongoing. It "aims to compare the clinical and cost-effectiveness of decompressive craniectomy versus craniotomy for the management of adult head-injured patients undergoing evacuation of an acute subdural hematoma (ASDH)."[33]

Surgical Procedure

In our example case, a unilateral left decompressive hemicraniectomy was accomplished. The patient, under general anesthesia, is placed in a supine position, with head turned to the contralateral side and placed on a horseshoe headrest or stabilized with a Mayfield clamp. The patient is then appropriately prepped and draped. Fast delimitation of the sagittal midline prior to draping can help avoid injury to the superior sagittal sinus, particularly in the trauma setting.

The neurosurgeon performed a left "trauma flap" incision, which is typically made as wide as possible for broad exposure, here encompassing the ipsilateral fronto-temporo-parietal region, passing at a minimum of approximately 2 cm lateral to the midline. A conventional question mark technique (used in this case) or a large "n"-shaped technique may be used for the incision.[34]

Fracture lines extending from parietal bone into temporal bone were visualized. The surgeon performed a left fronto-temporo-parietal craniectomy, partially incorporating fractures in the ipsilateral temporal bone in this case. The incision was made through the subcutaneous tissue, and the temporalis muscle was carefully dissected down to the zygoma. The temporal bone was removed until the middle fossa was decompressed; the dura is generally tense at this time. A durotomy was made in a semilunar fashion and based inferiorly.

The bone was not replaced because the brain usually appears swollen during the intervention. Surgicel and FloSeal matrix were used with meticulousness for hemostasis. A dural substitute (e.g., DuraGen, DuraSeal) was then applied (duraplasty), which would help during subsequent scalp dissection in case of eventual cranioplasty. A wound subgaleal drain was inserted on half suction. Vicryl sutures (e.g., 3-0) to galea and staples (or nylon sutures) to skin were applied for closure.[32,35]

Pivot Points

- In cases of fractures crossing the dural sinuses, the craniectomy is deliberately not extended posteriorly to avoid them. Inadvertently approaching the region can increase risk of sinus hemorrhage and occlusion.
- The surgeon should liaise with the neuroanesthesia team throughout the procedure and ask for hypoventilation and mannitol, which can lead to improvement in swelling.
- In this context, the brain should be further assessed intraoperatively for regional bleeding (e.g., an area of contusion at the left temporal lobe).

Aftercare

The patient was transferred back to the NCCU with continued ICP management. If ICP rises, a repeat scan is indicated; otherwise a postoperative follow-up scan 24 hours later can be arranged. The wound drain is generally removed at 24 h post-craniectomy, and staples are usually removed at 10–14 days post-craniectomy. If there is intracranial hypertension despite maximum medical therapy and previous decompressive hemicraniectomy, an EVD can be inserted (as was done in this case), provided the lateral ventricles are visible on CT, to help reduce intracranial volume further, even in the absence of hydrocephalus.

Full informed consent from next of kin was obtained. An EVD can be placed in the operative theater with a frontal linear incision (here on the right, to the nondominant lobe) behind and medial to a triple bolt around Kocher's point and a 4 mm burr hole. A CSF sample was sent to microbiology for analysis. Upon reversal of ICP control measures, a CO_2 challenge can be indicated to assess the patient's intracranial compliance (which is usually poor in intracranial hypertension) and to gauge the tolerance of de-escalation in ICP control measures. With the patient's clinical improvement, all parenchymal monitors can be removed at the same time upon discussion with the NCCU.

Complications and Management

A craniectomy is not a benign procedure and carries multiple risks including infection, new-onset hydrocephalus, subdural hygroma from perturbance of CSF dynamics, and vascular injury to the venous vasculature (especially cortical veins).[36] Moreover, a cranioplasty will need to be arranged to restore the skull's integrity and appearance on recovery. There is still no definitive evidence that a cranioplasty leads to improvement in functional outcomes, and its optimal timing (early vs. late) remains controversial.

Two serious posttraumatic complications to consider in our example case are presented in the Complications Pearls.[37–45]

Oral Boards Review: Complications Pearls

- *Sinking skin flap syndrome* (SSFS), also termed *syndrome of the trephined*, is a delayed and potentially disastrous complication of craniectomy due to a negative pressure gradient, with atmospheric pressure greater than ICP. SSFS classically presents with a sunken appearance of the skin overlying the skull defect and severe orthostatic headache. If left untreated, SSFS can lead to paradoxical brain herniation, coma, and death.
  - Paradoxical herniation from SSFS is a neurocritical care emergency. Management in the NCCU includes promptly stopping all measures to decrease ICP (e.g., clamping the EVD) and starting measures to increase ICP, for example putting the patient in the Trendelenburg position and administering IV fluid boluses. Cranioplasty constitutes definitive treatment for this disease in the absence of paradoxical herniation.
- *Cerebral venous sinus thrombosis* (CVST) following head trauma, which the example patient ultimately developed, is an underdiagnosed entity which can lead to devastating neurological sequelae. Patients typically present with headaches, focal deficits, seizures, encephalopathy, and/or isolated intracranial hypertension. Skull fractures, particularly if overlying a venous sinus, appear to be a predisposing factor to CSVT after closed head trauma. The surgeon should be aware of the presence of prothrombotic risk factors, either genetic (e.g., factor V Leiden mutation) or acquired (e.g., pregnancy, malignancy, use of oral contraceptives). Suspicion for CVST usually warrants urgent neuroimaging with venography; MRI with MRV is preferred due to improved sensitivity over CT with CTV, but the latter remains an option if MRV is not readily available.
  - Anticoagulation remains the main therapeutic option to consider for CVST; select case reports and case series show overall improved outcomes with anticoagulation treatment. However, the risks of therapeutic anticoagulation for posttraumatic CSVT, especially with concurrent intraaxial hemorrhages, are not well reported. Follow-up MRV or CTV can help assess the degree of sinus recanalization. Further prospective studies are necessary to better profile the course of this condition.

Evidence and Outcomes

The patient was discharged to the ward post-injury, with active rehabilitation and neuropsychology follow-up. This patient remained in posttraumatic amnesia on the ward, with full resolution at 6 weeks. The surgeon should collaborate with the neuropsychology and neurorehabilitation service to delineate the patient's profile of cognitive functioning on the ward if possible.

RESCUEicp showed a mortality rate of approximately 30.4% and a favorable outcome (defined in trial as GOS-E of 1–3: good recovery to upper severe disability) rate of 45.4% at 12 months in the DC group versus approximately 52.0% and approximately 32.4%, respectively, in the medical management group. ICP control was overall better in the DC group than in the medical management group. However, 37.2% of patients in the medical management group underwent DC after further deterioration. No "as-treated" analysis was reported in the study.[31]

Prognostic Models in TBI

Corticosteroid Randomization After Significant Head Injury (CRASH) and International Mission for Prognosis and Analysis of Clinical Trials in Traumatic Brain Injury (IMPACT) are two important prognostic models using admission patient characteristics to predict mortality and unfavorable outcome in sTBI patients.[46,47] These mathematical models were applied to specific population data and do not consider the patients' clinical course and interventions received. Thus, they cannot be accurately used for an individual patient.[48] Attention to each patient's clinical progress and particularities on a continual basis, using MMM among other tools, is a path to individualized care and improved therapeutic decisions.

References

1. Biffl WL, Moore EE, Offner PJ, et al. Optimizing screening for blunt cerebrovascular injuries. *Am J Surg.* 1999;178(6):517–522.
2. Watanabe K, Kida W. Images in clinical medicine. Battle's sign. *N Engl J Med.* 2012;367(12):1135.
3. Cohen-Inbar O, Kachel A, Levi L, Zaaroor M. Vaccination as primary prevention? The effect of anti-pneumococcal vaccination on the outcome of patients suffering traumatic skull base fractures. *J Neurosurg Sci.* 2017;61(3):245–255.
4. Hedberg AL, Pauksens K, Enblad P, et al. Pneumococcal polysaccharide vaccination administered early after neurotrauma or neurosurgery. *Vaccine.* 2017;35(6):909–915.
5. National Health Service. Patient group direction for Pneumovax II (23-valent pneumococcal vaccine [PPV]). In England PH, ed. London: National Health Service; 2014.
6. Smielewski P, Lavinio A, Timofeev I, et al. ICM+, a flexible platform for investigations of cerebrospinal dynamics in clinical practice. *Acta Neurochirurgica Suppl.* 2008;102:145–151.
7. Moberg. CNS Monitor. 2018; https://www.moberg.com/products/cns-monitor.
8. Anandic Medical Systems. BedMasterEx. 2018; https://www.bedmaster.net/en/products/bedmasterex.
9. Mokri B. The Monro-Kellie hypothesis: applications in CSF volume depletion. *Neurology.* 2001;56(12):1746–1748.
10. Brain Trauma Foundation. Guidelines for the Management of Severe Traumatic Brain Injury. Brain Trauma Foundation;2016.

11. Chesnut RM, Temkin N, Carney N, et al. A trial of intracranial-pressure monitoring in traumatic brain injury. *N Engl J Med.* 2012;367(26):2471–2481.

12. Hutchinson PJ, Kolias AG, Czosnyka M, Kirkpatrick PJ, Pickard JD, Menon DK. Intracranial pressure monitoring in severe traumatic brain injury. *Br Med J.* 2013;346:f1000.

13. Donnelly J, Budohoski KP, Smielewski P, Czosnyka M. Regulation of the cerebral circulation: bedside assessment and clinical implications. *Crit Care (London, England).* 2016;20(1):129.

14. Depreitere B, Guiza F, Van den Berghe G, et al. Pressure autoregulation monitoring and cerebral perfusion pressure target recommendation in patients with severe traumatic brain injury based on minute-by-minute monitoring data. *J Neurosurg.* 2014;120(6):1451–1457.

15. Steiner LA, Czosnyka M, Piechnik SK, et al. Continuous monitoring of cerebrovascular pressure reactivity allows determination of optimal cerebral perfusion pressure in patients with traumatic brain injury. *Crit Care Med.* 2002;30(4):733–738.

16. Liu X, Maurits NM, Aries MJH, et al. Monitoring of optimal cerebral perfusion pressure in traumatic brain injured patients using a multi-window weighting algorithm. *J Neurotrauma.* 2017;34(22):3081–3088.

17. CPPOpt Research Team. CPPOpt guided therapy: Assessment of target effectiveness (COGITATE). 2018.

18. Aries MJ, Czosnyka M, Budohoski KP, et al. Continuous determination of optimal cerebral perfusion pressure in traumatic brain injury. *Crit Care Med.* 2012;40(8):2456–2463.

19. Integra LifeSciences Corporation. Integra Licox® Brain Tissue Oxygen Monitoring System. 2018; http://occ.integralife.com/index.aspx?redir=detailproduct&Product=756&ProductName=Integra%AE%20Licox%AE%20Brain%20Tissue%20Oxygen%20Monitoring%20System%20%28LCX02%29&ProductLineName=Brain%20Tissue%20O2%20Monitoring&ProductLineID=10&PA=neurosurgeon.

20. Raumedic AG. Measurement of oxygen partial pressure in the brain. 2018; https://www.raumedic.com/neuromonitoring/neuro-icu/oxygen-partial-pressure/.

21. Okonkwo DO, Shutter LA, Moore C, et al. Brain oxygen optimization in severe traumatic brain injury phase-II: A phase II randomized trial. *Crit Care Med.* 2017;45(11):1907–1914.

22. NIH SIREN Emergencies Trials Network. Brain oxygen optimization in severe TBI Phase-3. 2018; https://siren.network/clinical-trials/boost-3.

23. MDialysis. ISCUSflex Microdialysis Analyzer. 2018; http://www.mdialysis.com/analyzers/iscusflex-for-point-of-care.

24. Timofeev I, Czosnyka M, Carpenter KL, et al. Interaction between brain chemistry and physiology after traumatic brain injury: Impact of autoregulation and microdialysis catheter location. *J Neurotrauma.* 2011;28(6):849–860.

25. Hutchinson PJ, Jalloh I, Helmy A, et al. Consensus statement from the 2014 International Microdialysis Forum. *Intens Care Med.* 2015;41(9):1517–1528.

26. Andrews PJ, Sinclair HL, Rodriguez A, et al. Hypothermia for intracranial hypertension after traumatic brain injury. *N Engl J Med.* 2015;373(25):2403–2412.

27. Lewis SR, Evans DJ, Butler AR, Schofield-Robinson OJ, Alderson P. Hypothermia for traumatic brain injury. *Cochrane Database Syst Rev.* 2017;9:Cd001048.

28. Cooper DJ, Nichol AD, Bailey M, et al. Effect of early sustained prophylactic hypothermia on neurologic outcomes among patients with severe traumatic brain injury: The POLAR randomized clinical trial. *JAMA.* 2018.

29. Minton MD, Stirt JA, Bedford RF, Haworth C. Intracranial pressure after atracurium in neurosurgical patients. *Anesth Analg.* 1985;64(11):1113–1116.

30. Ward S, Weatherley BC. Pharmacokinetics of atracurium and its metabolites. *Br J Anaesth.* 1986;58 Suppl 1:6s–10s.

31. Hutchinson PJ, Kolias AG, Timofeev IS, et al. Trial of decompressive craniectomy for traumatic intracranial hypertension. *N Engl J Med.* 2016;375(12):1119–1130.

32. Quinn TM, Taylor JJ, Magarik JA, Vought E, Kindy MS, Ellegala DB. Decompressive craniectomy: technical note. *Acta Neurologica Scandinavica.* 2011;123(4):239–244.

33. Rescue-ASDH Research Team. Rescue-ASDH. 2018; http://www.rescueasdh.org/.

34. Yang HS, Hyun D, Oh CH, Shim YS, Park H, Kim E. A faster and wider skin incision technique for decompressive craniectomy: n-Shaped incision for decompressive craniectomy. *Korean J Neurotrauma.* 2016;12(2):72–76.

35. Huang X, Wen L. Technical considerations in decompressive craniectomy in the treatment of traumatic brain injury. *Int J Med Sci.* 2010;7(6):385–390.

36. Nasi D, Gladi M, Di Rienzo A, et al. Risk factors for post-traumatic hydrocephalus following decompressive craniectomy. *Acta Neurochirurgica.* 2018;160(9):1691–1698.

37. Akins PT, Guppy KH. Sinking skin flaps, paradoxical herniation, and external brain tamponade: A review of decompressive craniectomy management. *Neurocrit Care.* 2008;9(2):269–276.

38. Jeyaraj P. Importance of early cranioplasty in reversing the "syndrome of the trephine/motor trephine syndrome/sinking skin flap syndrome." *J Maxillofac Oral Surg.* 2015;14(3):666–673.

39. Crimmins TJ, Rockswold GL, Yock DH, Jr. Progressive posttraumatic superior sagittal sinus thrombosis complicated by pulmonary embolism. Case report. *J Neurosurg.* 1984;60(1):179–182.

40. Giladi O, Steinberg DM, Peleg K, et al. Head trauma is the major risk factor for cerebral sinus-vein thrombosis. *Thrombosis Res.* 2016;137:26–29.

41. Ghuman MS, Salunke P, Sahoo SK, Kaur S. Cerebral venous sinus thrombosis in closed head trauma: A call to look beyond fractures and hematomas! *J Emergencies, Trauma, Shock.* 2016;9(1):37–38.

42. Grangeon L, Gilard V, Ozkul-Wermester O, et al. Management and outcome of cerebral venous thrombosis after head trauma: A case series. *Rev Neurol (Paris).* 2017;173(6):411–417.

43. Matsushige T, Nakaoka M, Kiya K, Takeda T, Kurisu K. Cerebral sinovenous thrombosis after closed head injury. *J Trauma.* 2009;66(6):1599–1604.

44. Oudeman EA, De Witt Hamer PC. Neurological picture. Successful outcome after traumatic rupture and secondary thrombosis of the superior sagittal sinus. *J Neurol Neurosurg Psychiatry.* 2013;84(10):1148–1149.

45. Saposnik G, Barinagarrementeria F, Brown RD, Jr., et al. Diagnosis and management of cerebral venous thrombosis: A statement for healthcare professionals from the American Heart Association/American Stroke Association. *Stroke.* 2011;42(4):1158–1192.

46. Perel P, Arango M, Clayton T, et al. Predicting outcome after traumatic brain injury: Practical prognostic models based on large cohort of international patients. *Br Med J.* 2008;336(7641):425–429.

47. Roozenbeek B, Lingsma HF, Lecky FE, et al. Prediction of outcome after moderate and severe traumatic brain injury: External validation of the International Mission on Prognosis and Analysis of Clinical Trials (IMPACT) and Corticoid Randomisation After Significant Head injury (CRASH) prognostic models. *Crit Care Med.* 2012;40(5):1609–1617.

48. Han J, King NK, Neilson SJ, Gandhi MP, Ng I. External validation of the CRASH and IMPACT prognostic models in severe traumatic brain injury. *J Neurotrauma.* 2014;31(13):1146–1152.

Index

For the benefit of digital users, indexed terms that span two pages (e.g., 52–53) may, on occasion, appear on only one of those pages.